TOGETHER ON OUR OWN

a novel

ELIANA MEGERMAN

EM Lit Press

Cover Design and Formatting by Damonza

In loving memory of my father,
Charles Megerman aka The Wizard

CHAPTER 1

UNLESS YOU'VE SHOWN up for your 7:00 a.m. shift at 7:00 p.m., you might not understand. The shared scattering of sunlight across the sky can make dawn indistinguishable from dusk. My pursuit of the study of medicine was meant to provide firmer ground, but the grounds were now shifting as the wind blew the sand away. It was in this fragile state of mind, nearing the end of the third year of an emergency medicine residency and struggling under the perpetually changing work hours, the crush of patients, the infinite reading assignments and the growing sense of isolation, that I learned about my hospital's plan to roll out a beta version of a new AI program that was meant to improve our skills as physicians. I was nodding off in the back row of a darkened classroom, having spent the previous night in the neuro ICU caring for an unfortunate gentleman in his sixties who'd presented to the ER unable to speak. His face drooped on one side, and he could not raise his left arm. Was he scared? Did he understand when we consented him to receive the clot busters that would travel through his blood stream and break up the clot in his middle cerebral artery? Or like the gray matter of his brain that was quickly melting away, had we landed in a gray zone in which he did not understand, and had to rely on his family to make the decision. Did they have his best interests at heart when they urged us to fill the syringe and push?

Hours later when he was unresponsive, and we informed his family that the clot busters had worked a little too well, that he was bleeding out in his brain, how did they feel about their decision? Had they really known his wishes? Faced with a future of dependence and aphasia, would he have rolled the dice with death? And what now? *Do Everything* was often the mantra. But what was everything when we'd landed with a brain bleed in the middle of the night in a formerly functional man? As I drifted and the lecturer droned on, the patient's twisted face flashed before me, until I heard the words "flexible," "efficient," and "purpose." My eyes snapped open, and my skin began to tingle, as I was overcome with an itch that spread from the soles of my feet to the back of my eyeballs. No amount of shuffling or blinking could release that powerful itch. As the administrator in front buzzed along with his flashy PowerPoint presentation, trying to convince us that the AI system was for our benefit, I knew it was not. I knew immediately that it would not provide more flexibility, efficiency and purpose, but like all the mandatory efficiency tools, would require my being flexible to incorporate a system thought up by those not involved in patient care. This AI system would likely not mean more efficiency, but rather more face time in front of a screen and less facing the actual patient. And I knew with deep certainty that it was not to provide more purpose to the resident doctors who were giving up nights, weekends and holidays for the privilege of caring for others. No, this could only be to streamline and benefit the administrator standing in front of the room. When he said the word authentic, the bile rose to the back of my throat, and I stifled a scream.

I cast my gaze around the room checking to see if the other residents were hearing the same alarms I was. The bells were ringing in my ears, yet they looked calm and focused, taking notes. It seems obvious that I should have gone for help. Drowning as I was in my excessive workload, exhaustion, and shrinking under the heavy responsibilities, getting help should have been the right thing to do. But the culture in medicine is such that those of us who have dedicated our lives to stomping out disease must conduct ourselves in such a way as if sickness is a myth or fantasy that only impacts others. We, the healers, dwell only in the world of perfect health. Like so many values that can butt up against each other, the oath we take while still students: First Do No Harm, clashes mightily with the underlying message: Physician, heal thyself. Admitting weakness is admitting defeat. A flu-like illness had knocked me out the year before but when I asked my senior if a fever of one hundred and three meant I should go home, she gave me a look. A look that I didn't need to put through any translation app because the meaning was so clear. There could be no fever, no cough, no illness that would stand in between me and my duties that day. We'd been told of a surgery resident who gave birth hours after finishing a case. The twinges of pain on her face were not warning signs about a young woman pushed to the brink, standing for hours in front of a splayed open body. No, she was a hero who hadn't let the insignificant needs of her personal life and her body interfere with her obligations at the hospital. Even as they told us that we could always ask for help, the unwritten rule was to never, ever, under any circumstance, ask for help.

The prevailing culture was and always had been that suffering was something done best in silence. Had that laboring resident groaned as her body contracted, or had she swallowed the sounds? After graduating from medical school, we were required to obtain a medical license. We would complete the required forms annually for the rest of our lives first to obtain and then renew our medical licenses. The forms varied slightly from state to state but were very specific when they asked about mental health. Had we been to a psychologist? Had we needed any form of treatment? The answer, in order to expedite license approval, was "no." Any "yes" answer required clarification and explanation, because why would any physician require help?

There'd been a suicide the year before I started. We didn't overlap, but when I heard the rumors (and there were many), I remembered meeting her the day I'd interviewed with the program that I ultimately chose. She was the chief resident, and we'd stood in awe as we watched her running a trauma code with the trauma team on a young kid who'd been shot in the back. With blood spurting out of tubes as they cracked open his chest, they'd tried valiantly to do the impossible. She squeezed his heart in her gloved hands, trying to defy death. She did not succeed. Did her shoulders sag a little as she tore off her blue plastic gown and tossed it in the trash before exiting the trauma bay to give us a tour of the emergency department? Was there a shadow over her face before she turned on the smile and greeted us, regaling us with her tales of life in the ER? But she was good and tidy and didn't put her needs above the system.

Afterwards, my training program implemented a mental health seminar. Attendance was mandatory. During that mandatory hour, they were explicit that anyone who needed help should immediately turn to the leadership. It was an absolute top priority for the hospital. Priority number one. What they weren't so explicit about was what would happen if you turned to them for help. Would they hold your position if you needed some time off? Would your circumstance be kept confidential, or like every other word whispered in the hospital, would it quickly spread like an old-fashioned game of telephone with the details changing slightly with each telling? Depending on your social standing, those dynamic details would alter to elicit either sympathy or more often, harsh and swift judgment. If the chief resident hadn't been comfortable going to them, who were we, brand new peons at the bottom of the totem pole, to try to seek out care? Sickness was only for the weak, that much was understood.

And so, as my sleep became more ephemeral, as the recurring thoughts in my head got louder, I knew the only course of action was to try harder to bury them. Lying awake at night, I would panic thinking about a confused elderly patient I'd seen that day. I'd chalked up her low-grade fever to a urinary tract infection, but in retrospect, was it inflammation of her brain? Had I missed a subtle presentation of encephalitis and now that sharp grandmother with her cluster of pearls, and ruby red lips would disintegrate as the virus devoured her mind? I wanted to call her and ask how she was doing, but it was 02:00 a.m. Even if she answered, the middle of the night phone call wouldn't explain any confusion on her end. And it wasn't as if I had her personal contact information at the ready. It would require calling into the ER and asking one of my colleagues to look her up. I could almost hear their accusation: *You didn't do an LP on an elderly patient with fever and altered mental status?*

The week before, I'd texted a colleague working the night shift to ask about a patient with chest pain. I'd discharged him, but as the night grew darker, my mind couldn't rest. Had I missed an aortic dissection? Was he at home now, clutching his chest and losing consciousness as his aorta ripped open and leaked out the contents of his life? I could see his wife calling an ambulance, but it would be too late by the time he reached the ER. My colleagues would pound on his chest, they'd force a tube down his throat to breathe for him, but no amount of pumping or pushing would restart his heart. Not after my fatal mistake. I waited until daybreak to call him; I tried convincing my disgruntled mind to sleep until that time. He answered on the fifth ring. He was fine if a little perturbed by the early morning wake up call.

As the administrator droned on about the benefits of the new AI system, I grew increasingly agitated. My dreams of medicine had not included computers and electronic data input. For every moment I spent with a patient, I spent four minutes clicking through screens with an increasing number of documentation requirements. Not for better patient care, but for meeting the needs of the complex and multiplying administrative bureaucracy. My fellow residents seemed immune to it. Though we'd come at it from different backgrounds mostly. There wasn't a new technology they didn't embrace. Instead of sitting at the patient's bedside making eye contact, they stared at screens and compared graphics. Forget listening to a patient's history; after rapid fire introductions, their hands were on the ultrasound probe, peeking in and seeing what ailed them.

I was older than most of the other residents. They'd more or less been on a straight trajectory from high school. Some of them middle school. Everything in their lives had been focused on one goal. After college, unsure which direction I should take my undergraduate journalism degree, I answered an ad to teach English in Panama. My Spanish was decent, but after six months abroad I was fluent and answered another ad. This time for a clerical position at a clinic. Though I had hardly the skills of a candy striper, the senior physician at the clinic, noting my interest, took me under his wing. I accompanied him on rounds in the hospital, home visits and even a few births. He worked with very limited resources, an old portable ultrasound that had been donated by a visiting church group was his most used tool, but he held his patients' hands. He spoke with the woman whose knee kept swelling up, he felt the spine of the day laborer with low back pain, he palpated the abdomen of the teenager who vomited after eating spicy foods, and he reflected on their conditions. His diagnostic skills, which I marveled at in real time, I later learned were a vanishing skill. I watched as doctors examined patients without so much as touching them. As the technology expanded, my colleagues were eager to get the Star Trek wand of the future in their hand that could tell them immediately what was wrong with the patient. Like a modern mechanic running computer diagnostics on the car. It didn't all feel like progress. It felt like a growing crevice between me and the patients I'd signed up to care for. Underneath the wearying number of them and the ever-expanding list of forms and boxes I needed to tick and click, I had trouble imagining how the AI system would help.

Having recently turned thirty-one (a milestone somehow more significant than thirty had seemed) I entered a new period of my life. I became mired in self-doubt. Instead of finding more confidence and self-assuredness, I became almost confused in questioning my competence. As if I'd entered a new universe where one plus one could be three if I only thought about it more. Considered a different angle. In an argument over the color of my eyes (hazel grey) and with no mirror in sight, I could almost become convinced that they were blue. Or had been blue at some point, maybe? Facts slipped through my fingers even on issues I was certain about. I double and triple checked patients' X-rays as the images blurred together from previous films and blood tests.

Friends from college bragged about promotions, weddings, engagements—one even had a baby—whereas I was still training and swallowed up with menial tasks. And my love life was a series of bad dates and no starts. My last serious boyfriend had been a Peace Corps volunteer in Panama. When he broke up with me, he'd explained his dreams and aspirations, which didn't include marriage or a *conventional* life. He'd used the word conventional in a derogatory tone, as if reserved for lesser people. Lesser people like me, who was moving back to the United States to begin medical school. One year later, as I sat memorizing neural pathways and peptide complexes, I saw his wedding pictures on social media. His wife, stunning in her corset-style, A-line, ivory gown, was beautiful in every *conventional* way. From my cyber-stalking I discovered that she was a software engineer at a large tech firm. I tried remembering the way he'd chewed his nails and left clusters of them dispersed on our breakfast table, rather than the specific flex of his forearms when he rolled up his sleeves to fix our ever-leaking kitchen sink.

That evening, I was supposed to go on a date. As soon as the AI lecture was over, I had forty-eight hours off and away from the hospital. I checked my phone; my time off had already dwindled to forty-six hours. The speaker opened to questions. I inhaled quickly and hoped that my fellow residents would remain silent. Those of us after a night shift were desperate to get out but a few people in the room were on very demanding rotations and surely wanted to stretch the time that they were seated in the auditorium drinking coffee, and not getting badgered and pimped by their attendings. Pimping or asking increasingly detailed and complicated questions about the patient's presentation, sickness and treatment was a standard method of teaching. Eventually, most of us got used to the spotlight, but occasionally every crumb of information that you'd memorized and tucked away for future use was obliterated by the intense pressure of all peers in your group staring you down and waiting for your answer. Some attendings were nice and guided you in a learning direction, and some pounced at the first hint of indecision, and like a mortar and pestle, ground the medical student or intern down to a mushy paste. True to form, one of the gunners sitting in the front row asked a question that had several possible answers and forced another eight minutes of the meeting.

After we were dismissed, I snuck into the physicians' lounge hoping to scrounge up breakfast without being spotted by anyone who could assign me a task. Technically, our "off time" was mandated by the government, but in practice there were many ways around the mandate. Usually in the form of being assigned an asinine task that would "only take a minute." Whatever they'd served for breakfast that morning was mostly gone, so I swiped a clementine and a yogurt. A tray of muffins sat in the center of the buffet. Each muffin was oddly dissected as if a surgical team on a diet had swooped in. Three blueberry muffin halves were left behind, evidence of the psychos I worked with. Why did they pretend that someone was going to take the half they'd left behind? And if that half was so valuable, why hadn't one of them taken a half instead of cutting into a fresh muffin?

Sapna, a third-year surgery resident entered the lounge. I pointed at the tray.

"Savages," she muttered as she rolled her eyes. The dark grey circles under her eyes seemed deeper than usual, though her Kohl rimmed eyes were hardly smudged. I'd seen Sapna in several precarious situations and never once seen her without perfectly lined lids.

"I'm like a hobbit today, back for my second breakfast," she said as she scanned the remnants.

"Slim pickings," I replied.

She picked up a muffin half, peeled off the wrapper and took a bite as she popped a coffee pod into the coffee maker.

Pointing her chin towards the backpack casually slung over my shoulder, she gave a half grin.

"You outta here?"

We weren't covering the same service, so she couldn't hurt me. Plus, Sapna was thoughtful and kind; she wouldn't dump work on someone trying to get out. We'd gone to a party together a few months ago, and I'd gotten a little too drunk. Even though she was having fun, she left with me.

"I have two whole days off. I even have a date tonight."

"First date or second?"

"Why do you assume it's only a first or second date? No possibility in your mind that this could be number five or six?"

Leaning back against the counter, she held the coffee cup between her hands and blew on the surface. Her long black hair cascaded down her shoulders. "First of all, if you were going on a fifth date, I would have already heard about him."

I nodded.

"But more importantly…" She stopped as she took a halting sip of her coffee. "If you'd met a man that held more appeal than sitting in your pajamas watching TV, I'd see it on your face."

"Am I that transparent?" I asked as I tightened my grip on my backpack strap.

She narrowed her eyes and cocked her head to the side as if sizing me up. "You already know my theory."

Sapna had theories on so many things, chief among them was her theory on the multitude of personality disorders we were forced to work with. On that count, I mostly agreed with her. Her strong opinions and stubborn streak were part of what made her tough enough to push through a predominantly male-dominated specialty. Growing up, she'd spent summers in India visiting family and giving her parents a chance to eat the foods of their childhood. She told me once that the poverty she'd seen as they traveled around was unlike anything she'd seen in the United States. Even as a young child, she'd intuited that one or two twists of fate could have landed her in a very different situation. And so whatever happened in her life, she felt that she had not experienced true suffering. No matter if someone tried to drill her down with their pimping questions, if they mistook her for a hospital janitor, if they excluded her from a social event, it didn't touch her. She was almost robotic in her ability to deflect, as if she'd built a forcefield around her. I'd seen that forcefield protect her in the male dominated surgery world.

Knowing Sapna, it might have been an actual forcefield. In addition to being wicked smart, she was also tall, lithe and gorgeous. Whereas most people that looked like her were hanging out with the cool kids, her strong passion for Star Wars and seeming obliviousness to her own looks had her always choosing the nerds. Maybe they'd built a forcefield for themselves to protect them from the way of the world. It's probably why we got along. She wasn't one to cower, and she had her eye on the prize. It helped that both of her parents were physicians: A cardiologist and a dermatologist who routinely discussed interesting cases at the dinner table with their children. Sapna's brother was a radiology resident at a different hospital system. He was handsome, but she never introduced us. She and her brother were expected to marry other Indian Americans. Her parents had a roster of potential marriage candidates. This was another issue she had strong opinions about, since she'd been seriously dating a non-Indian resident in the vascular surgery program for over a year. As strong willed as she was, she hadn't yet broken the news to her parents.

Her theory on my love life was that I was seduced by the allure of a perfect companion who didn't exist. That the constant swiping on apps and seemingly endless supply of candidates meant I would never take the leap because someone more appealing might be my next swipe. She offered this idea as if men were beating down my door, as if I'd had multiple offers that I'd refused, as if the men on the other side of the swipe weren't doing the same thing, meeting me with one eye on the next possible better candidate. Sapna was right. Part of my indecisiveness was spilling over into my romantic life. I tried managing my expectations, but humans were messy and needy, and half the time didn't call you when they said they would.

"This guy seems different. We connected a bit already; I think we're going to have a good time."

She shook her head in disbelief. "Let me know how it goes."

I turned to leave and noticed a resident sitting at a cubicle dictating. When had he walked in? Had he been there the entire time? His badge identified him as a physical medicine and rehab doctor. The term was a mouthful, so they referred to themselves as PM&R, which I think most patients thought was a fake specialty when they heard it. As if their doctor was a specialist in M&M candies or rest and relaxation. I knew most of the rehab residents from my neuro rotations, and I would have remembered him, with his mop of wavy black hair, olive skin and chocolate brown eyes. I tried slinking by, but he turned and gave a lopsided grin as he pointed to his muffin, circling it to show that it had not been cut in half.

❧

Later that night as I readied myself for my date, I tried tempering my expectations. Sapna was wrong on that account. I didn't reject these men outright, but often it was like meeting someone from another planet. Almost like a prisoner, when I had furlough from the hospital, I often found interactions with people not training at the hospital to be fraught with misunderstanding. We spoke different languages, and my preoccupation with bodily fluids and gallows humor could make me seem callous and awkward.

When they said they wanted to hear the sickest thing I'd seen, they never meant it. They weren't interested in maggots in ear canals, feet so rotten and macerated that socks nearly peeled blackened toes off as I removed them. Dates took a definite turn for the worse if I brought up growths oozing pus or eating through chest walls. And no one wanted to hear about the four-hundred-pound man who'd choked on a peanut butter sandwich. I'd responded with the rest of the code team to the overhead pages and found him on the floor. An intern jumped on his chest to start chest compressions, and it became clear we would not be able to hoist this man back onto his bed. I intubated him on the floor, digging my way through vomit and sticky peanut butter.

"Can you imagine your last meal being a stale hospital peanut butter sandwich?" My date didn't laugh the way the resident in the ICU had at 4:00 a.m. when I made the joke. I laughed too, after I'd stopped shaking, after we'd gotten a pulse back and transferred him to the intensive care unit.

"I suppose it's better than those dreadful turkey sandwiches you guys hand out in the ER," the resident had joked back. An hour later, the patient lost his pulse again. This time they couldn't get it back. It was like that. We could work so hard, scrambling on floors, pumping chests, inserting airways and yet death often outsmarted us at every turn. My dates didn't care for those stories. They wanted sterilized versions like they'd seen on television, not the wet and dank cases I was dealing with every day. Even the hedge fund manager, sparkling in his confidence and buttoned up cuffs, had squirmed in his seat when I told him about a man with a lightbulb in his rectum.

"But how did you get it out?" He visibly recoiled as he glanced at my hands and seemed to calculate where they had been and if we'd shaken hands when I arrived.

"He had to go to the operating room," I explained. But he was no longer listening, already scanning the restaurant for the quickest exit strategy and trying to remember which friend had introduced us so he could cross him off the Christmas card list.

I'd upped my strategy and now avoided mentioning anything involving bandages, pus or discomfort. I was considering making up a job for first dates. I sometimes did this on airplanes. That way I avoided hearing about my seatmate's rash or unexplained fatigue that their doctor couldn't figure out. Worse were their stories about malpractice, as if I wanted to hear my colleagues maligned in some way or remind myself that someone out there might be telling a story about me and my seeming indifference. A perfect career would be business or management that was vague enough not to elicit questions. A job that could remain undefined for our first few meetings, though I worried about when I would tell them. What if we did hit it off? There wouldn't be a proper time to explain that I'd lied about my career choice in order to make meeting me more palatable.

My last date hadn't gone well. We'd exchanged a series of increasingly flirty texts leading up to the date, so I was looking forward to meeting him. When I arrived at the bar he'd chosen, I was pleasantly surprised to find that he resembled his profile picture. As he swirled his drink and leaned a self-assured arm on the bar, he roped me into telling a hospital story. His sly grin disarmed me, but I still stuck to my new and wiser approach, avoiding any talk about weeping wounds or death. I focused on one of the elderly demented patients I'd taken care of during my Internal Medicine rotation.

Dolores had entered the hospital with a simple urine infection. (I caught myself as he raised his glass of beer to take a swig, and avoided mentioning the word urine.) Dolores was eighty years old and lived alone on relatively meager means. The admitting team thought that her altered mental status would improve after they treated the infection, but it turned out she'd been battling dementia for quite some time and none of her family wanted to take her in. Without a great insurance strategy and little savings, she was dependent on state funds to find a nursing home, which meant she was housed on the internal medicine ward until the social work team could find placement.

I mistook the look on his face to be one of interest, and

with that encouragement I continued on. Dolores was not what we referred to as "pleasantly demented." Those ladies were happy to sip their tea and pretend they were entertaining or telling jokes at a garden party. They might not answer any of your questions appropriately, but it was always with charm and a smile. They might compliment my shoes (black clogs, worn for comfort) or hair style, not appropriate in our particular setting, but they were pleasant nonetheless. There was a particular joy I experienced when one of these patients would tell a senior male attending that his haircut suited him.

Dolores was not pleasant, nor was she neutral. She was a slugger. And she was remarkably fast for her age and condition, even landing a few punches on an unsuspecting intern and a couple of the nurses. When the family of a roommate who'd received a black eye threatened to call the state, Dolores was moved to a single room. All of this—her age, her poverty, and her tendency towards violence—made placement in a nursing home more complicated. When her family visited (which was rare and brief), I tried to fish out what she had been like before the dementia. Had she always had the violent streak? But either my questions were not direct enough or they didn't want to say.

My date and I had met for drinks at a trendy club a few blocks from the hospital. The music was loud enough that I had to yell out certain parts. Between the buzz of my Vodka tonic, the pounding bass, and my shouting to be heard, I missed his facial cues that would have informed another person to change tacks. Mistaking his widening eyes for curiosity, I powered through about legislation, restraints and the paperwork involved in tying people to their beds. Letting her roam the hospital like a boxer throwing punches was hardly a viable option. Not only because there were staff and other patients to worry about, but because every swing she took made it less and less likely to find her placement. As a solution, most days Dolores was sedated with a cocktail not dissimilar to the ones we were currently drinking. Sedation led to its own series of complications, and we strove to avoid turning her into a version of some of our other patients waiting for placement. Those with tubes and diapers who were watered and changed every day without registering one sunset to the next.

"If you give a mouse a cookie," I said.

"You have mice in the hospital?" He looked incredulous.

It was at about that point I began to suspect that what I had mistaken for interest was actually horror. I gulped my drink and tried to recover the witty banter we'd experienced before meeting face-to-face. Our mutual interest in Jon Krakauer should have translated to an actual relationship. Many of my dates hadn't heard of the famous mountain climber and showed no interest in learning about his near-death experience climbing Mount Everest. But instead of cresting the mountain of first dates, I'd bungled my anchor and was slipping off the side of the cliff. I sent a quick text to Sapna hoping she could help me salvage the situation. In spite of her penchant for light sabers and jedi masters, she was very sharp about social matters.

> I think I freaked my date out with stories about tying Slugger down. SOS.

I hit send and waited for her instructions. His phone sat

face up on the bar and I heard a ding. I preferred keeping my phone in my bag and ignoring it on dates, but that didn't seem to be the norm. Whatever phone etiquette was meant to be on dates, I noted a general pattern. There were three types: those who kept their phone out of sight (preferred), those who kept it face down on the table (still good) and those who kept it face up or even in their hands. Unfortunately, in my experience, most guys kept it face up and glanced over with every buzz and beep, so that I was forced to not only be charming but to constantly compete with a low level, continuous distraction. Once or twice, I'd observed texts come in from other women on the dating app. Some men had the propriety to at least appear ashamed when that happened, but more than one had actually responded to those texts right in front of me. One had even made plans for later that night. It had me wondering how many texts I was receiving while the sender was on a date with someone else.

Immediately hearing his phone ding, after sending Sapna the text, I felt a sinking feeling. My grappling boots were losing all traction as the pebbles gathered and fell. I looked down at my screen. Instead of texting Sapna, I'd sent it directly to him. I hadn't noticed that I'd left our fun texting session open.

As he reached for his phone I scrambled for a solution. Something witty to salvage this avalanche. I toggled on the delete button but not before he'd read the text. It changed to *You Deleted This Message* in front of his eyes. He signaled for the check and thanked me for an "interesting" night. It was like slicing into an avocado only to discover the green interior had turned brown, and still in desperation trying a bite and having to spit it out along with hopes for the perfect bite.

"Maybe you *should* start telling people that you're a librarian," Sapna suggested the next day as we were grabbing lunch trays in the cafeteria trying to dissect the evening and the myriad ways it had exploded. "You certainly know enough about books."

"I think there's more to being a librarian than a love of reading," I said as I scooped some mashed potatoes onto my plate.

Sapna checked her watch as she stealthily strode through the cafeteria, procuring the limited healthy options that weren't visible to the rest of us. She was like a hospital food magician, able to pull fresh vegetables and whole grains out of a buffet line that held greasy burgers, French fries and chicken fingers for the rest of us. She'd learned early on in training to avoid large fatty meals before scrubbing in on a surgery. After inhaling a super-sized milkshake and nuggets, she was an hour into a three-hour surgery when she'd felt her stomach grumbling and growling. Unable to hold out, she let a silent fart loose in the room. One of the attendings had mistaken the overpowering smell of that rancid fart for nicked bowel, a feared and potentially deadly complication. As he announced his intention to "run the bowel" searching for their error, she'd had to admit in front of the entire room that she had passed gas. I'd yet to see her with another milkshake.

Tonight's date would be different. Having already swiped right on most of the possibilities, I'd needed to find a new dating app. Ads for this app began appearing in my social media feed weeks before, which only added to the feeling that my phone was listening to me. I understood intellectually about algorithms and targeted advertising, but it didn't explain conversations about obscure topics that suddenly appeared in my feed. The day after I'd forgotten about a pot of boiling eggs and found a scorched, smoky mess, I received an ad for "the perfect electric egg cooker." It could even poach eggs, which sent me down the rabbit hole of correct methods, a subject for which I had no interest and yet lost an evening to. My devices fed right into my growing obsession with microplastics. I switched to a metal water bottle, and glass food containers, but everywhere I looked I seemed to be consuming from or interacting with plastic. Was it safe to handle paper receipts? Apparently, those too were toxic. How had everything become toxic overnight? I thought longingly of Panama and the single ceramic coffee mug from which I drank almost everything.

Even though I was certain my devices were listening, they sometimes missed the big picture. I received several ads for a language app that would help me interact with the growing Spanish speaking population. I'd lived in Panama for years and spoke almost at mother tongue level. Take that!

So, it was with a bit of caution that I was trying this app. The algorithms knew both random intimate details about me and yet nothing at all. Plus, the culture of certain apps wasn't always apparent until after meeting the various candidates. Tonight's date wanted to go ice-skating. I pushed down my images of broken ankles and scalp lacerations and headed out with a good attitude. I would tell no medical tales, and I would go with the flow. I hoped. I'd last been ice skating at my friend Katy's twelfth birthday. She'd worn a glittering purple figure skating dress and I'd spent the rest of sixth grade dreaming of looking like Katy one day. In memory of that party, I pulled a light blue sweater top covered in sequins stripes from my closet but swapped it for a simple navy top and jeans.

When I arrived at the rink, I found him standing outside. Tall, curly brown hair, and a decent build. He smiled and waved. I wondered what it was like when people met on dates not having already seen photos of each other. Not having to measure the way the person actually looked against the way they presented themselves online. We exchanged pleasantries.

"Should we get out of here?" he asked.

I was momentarily confused. Was that new slang for should we go inside rent skates and proceed with our date, or did it have the same meaning it always had?

"Aren't we going to skate?" I asked, the blunder not yet apparent.

"Exactly," he nodded.

This did nothing to clear up my confusion.

"Was there another skating rink you wanted to try?" I asked.

He gave me a strange look and pulled his phone out, muttering something about the app and wasting his time. He scrolled to my profile and held it up to me as if seeing a picture of myself on his screen would help me understand the situation we currently found ourselves in. Standing outside of an ice-skating rink on a first date talking about leaving.

"This is a hook-up app."

I thought of my sparkling sequins sweater cast aside on my bed. How differently I would see it when I returned home, and how glad I was now that I had not worn it. An image of a trichomonas parasite swimming along under a microscope came to mind.

"I, um…"

He looked me up and down. "You thought we were actually going ice skating?" He asked in a way that was not unkind.

I nodded and took a step back, preventing further entanglement in a situation that I had completely misread.

"No worries. But it's not that kind of app."

I understood that now. And clearly. He waved again, though this time with less enthusiasm than when he had greeted me, and turned on his heel. I pulled my phone out and reread the series of texts we'd exchanged in a very different light. I then permanently deleted the app from my phone. So often I hesitated when asked if I was sure, did I really want to delete this message, app or contact information? The message sent flickering waves of panic through my system. What if I needed it again in the future, was it really forever irretrievable? How certain could we be what we might need in the future?

But this time, I was sure. Very sure.

CHAPTER 2

A WEEK LATER I had my first shift using the new AI technology. I tried to remember the highlights from the introductory talk that I'd mostly slept through. Phrases such as time-saving, increased accuracy, and more time with patients came to mind, but as they handed me and the other residents the fine print to sign, the project seemed more aligned with cost effectiveness and bottom lines. A buzz in the back of my brain, a sixth sense of sorts that had developed during my years studying journalism, grew louder. Quieting that buzz would entail reading through the pages of fine print instead of flipping past them. As I turned the first page of legalese, chewing away at my blue pen, my suspicions worsened. My interests were not what was being protected on these forms. The weight of the others in the room watching as I studied the forms descended upon me. A hush had fallen, and that worrying buzz morphed into a prickling on my neck as the sighs and whispers began. I was the only one who hadn't signed. How long could I let the illusion of control linger? A discomfiting realization, like a tiny seed sprouting, blossomed into full bloom under the weight of those stares, and I swallowed my concerns whole and scribbled away in blue ink on the dotted line.

Next, we were given two options: Carry a small tablet into each patient encounter or download the app to our phones and keep our phones on during patient encounters. As leery as I was about the project, I chose option one. Faced with voluntarily installing a listening device onto my cell phone seemed alarming at best. But I was the odd one out that morning. We were one of five hospitals in the region to pilot this technology and I noted that the rep came armed with only a small box of tablets. He looked at me funny when I gave my preference. It was only me and three other doctors that stood in line for the tablet. One was a surgical resident who had moved to the United States from China as a young child. On more than one occasion, I'd seen him snigger when residents complained about long hours and their rights being violated. Another was a radiology resident who was now doing a fellowship in interventional radiology. He had a swagger and ease about him that radiated confidence. Passing fishing line size wires through vessels to pull out clots or deploy tiny coils to stop bleeding required a certain boldness. I didn't know him well, but he was up to date on every latest gadget and technology and his presence in our small group of dissidents buoyed me. He was reviewing a CT angiogram on his phone when he looked up.

"I already downloaded the app onto my phone. Am I free to go?"

The rep smiled wide and shook his hand heartily. "I'll call you later."

"You bet," he answered. He winked as he strode away.

Winked! Such was his assuredness, and I wished I could spend a day in his shoes to recapture that feeling for myself. Perhaps that's how he felt when he looked at me, an ER resident. It required nerves of steel to tell a family it was okay to take their baby with fever home when at that very moment a life-threatening bacteria could be travelling through its bloodstream. Confidence was required to discharge a middle-aged man with crushing chest pain he thought was a heart attack, or a young woman with abdominal pain who was sure her condition was serious. I'd had that confidence once. Before the incident. Before my nerves had been melted down by my mistake. Now, the looks I got were tinged with anxiety, as if the error I'd made could be contagious. What would happen to his swagger the first time his wire accidentally pierced through a vessel, or he accidentally dislodged a clot and a patient's feet needed to be amputated?

As he left our group, the life preserver floated away, and I was once again a stone dropping down in endless waters. The third person waiting for the tablet was the rehab resident I'd seen in the lounge. The rep looked at our motley crew of three not with disdain, but with a look of concern rolled up in pity. As if we were that man on the beach throwing in one starfish at a time because it made a difference to *that* starfish, but he knew that the starfish were imaginary. I believe he realized that eventually we too would understand what was so clear to everyone else, but the starfish still seemed real to us. I looked over at the surgical resident, but he was reviewing notes for a surgery he was scheduled to scrub in on later that day. The rehab resident stepped forward.

"Now I know two things about you," he said as we waited

for our tablets. "You don't like people touching your baked goods, and you are hesitant to sign your privacy away."

"After all those microbiology classes we took, I'm surprised any of us eat anything other people have touched," I said. My cheeks flushed, as I wondered how much of my conversation with Sapna he'd overheard.

"We have to forget about most of the things we learn, or we couldn't function in the real world. Hazard is around every corner."

"I hope you haven't forgotten most of the things we learned," I countered. In contrast to me, he emanated serenity and as I absorbed his calmness, I leaned into the conversation. Perhaps he was thinking the same about me, magnetized by my calm exterior, unaware of the barrage of rapid-fire thoughts I was constantly fielding.

"*Touché.*"

"And privacy? The hospital is the worst. You don't even need words to start a rumor in this place. Thoughts alone are enough."

He chuckled. It was absurd to me that he seemed unaware of the investigation against me, given the strength of the rumor mill.

"To that point, I didn't realize you were in the lounge that day when I was talking to my friend," I said.

He drew two closed fingers across his lips.

"I'm Henry." He extended his hand, and we shook; his grip was firm and warm. He looked at me expectantly as I dropped my hand to my side. "I know both of those things about you, but I don't know your name."

Searching for my name, Henry managed to glance at my

badge without ogling my chest, an impressive feat. It was turned inward, so I reversed it and showed him. My ID picture was of a person who was spirited and hopeful. Sometimes I wished I could travel back and give her a few warnings, something to help keep her spirits up. But there were risks involved with that plan. Given enough warning, there could be unintended consequences. That and the inability to travel through time prevented me from further messing things up.

"Alex Galen. Nice to meet you."

"Alex Galen." A look of recognition crossed his face.

"I've heard it all, you don't have to make the connection."

"The connection?"

Years of people commenting on the name Galen, a Greek physician from the second century known as one of the founding fathers of medicine, had accustomed me to a certain response. It was a rare member of the medical community who could resist pointing out the coincidence. Those who refrained weren't holding back, but just hadn't paid enough attention to my name, as if they were baristas at coffee bars who could write whatever version of the real name they made up. Whether any of these medical students and doctors believed that it was news to me seemed unlikely. Unless they regarded me as a modern-day Rip Van Winkle, having woken up from a two-thousand-year sleep and only now learning about the original Galen. At this point in my medical career, it felt as if I had been responding to these comments for two millennia Though there was no proof of any relation, I was in good company. Galen was a man who fought the establishment, and firmly believed in the mind-body connection. He also believed that the human body consisted of four different liquids known as humor, and that illness was caused by an imbalance of our humors. Everyone smirked when they first heard the theory, but had we really progressed so much? As we rushed forward with our devices, were we so superior? I tried to imagine Galen now, being handed a tablet to listen in on his patient encounters and make him more cost-effective. Would he have embraced this changing landscape with its promises of less stress and burnout? Generally, when people comment on my name a simple nod and smile moved the conversation forward.

"The connection between me and Galen."

A puzzled look crossed his face and then it clicked. "Of course. *The* Galen. Humors and all that. We owe a lot to him."

"Who were you thinking of?"

"Alex like Alexander. There's a famous violinist."

"Alexandra actually, and I'm not up to date on famous violinists."

He waved his hand as if shooing a bug away. "As famous as a violin player can get."

"He's no Itzhak Perlman is what you're telling me."

"And you said you weren't up to date," he teased.

"He made a few appearances on Sesame Street. Can I get credit if I say Yo-Yo Ma, even though it's the cello?"

"I'll grant you ten points."

"We've only just met and already you're appealing to my competitive side."

"You're in good company there."

"Game on. I'll grant you fifty points for not commenting on my last name."

"Thank you. And now I know one more thing about you."

I raised an eyebrow.

"You're more generous than I am when handing out credits."

"You may be disappointed when you discover their worth."

He gave a sly grin. "I doubt it. I don't get the sense you give out points so easily."

I wasn't sure if it was meant as a compliment or a challenge of sorts.

"And why are famous violinists top of your mind?"

A look flashed across his eyes, but it was gone before I could classify it. He seemed to size me up and then he stuck out his hands. They trembled as he held them in front of me.

"I was a musician." He pulled his hands back. "Violin was a very important part of my life. I was one of *those* kids." He made a funny face, half mocking, half serious.

"A prodigy?"

He shrugged, but I detected no sense of superiority. Maybe it was like medicine. If you surrounded yourself with students who were always at the top of the class, it was easy to feel like a failure when you landed in the middle among them. Maybe he'd been in the top twenty prodigy children in the world, and since it wasn't in the top ten or even the coveted number one spot, he felt like a failure in his world. I took in his relaxed stance. Maybe he had been number one but despite years of adulation, he remained humble.

"I was very talented, but I worked very hard. Practicing eight hours a day was nothing. I toured around during high school and I went to Juilliard with the expectation of a professional career." He clasped his hands together and stretched his arms long. "In my senior year I developed a benign tremor."

He unclasped his hands and held them out for me again.

We watched his tremor almost as if it was not a part of his body.

"That's rough." It was an understatement to say the least.

He put his hands in his pockets and rocked back. "It took some time to adjust."

"So, medicine was your backup plan? I was impressed enough when you said Juilliard. I imagine you're popular at dinner parties." As soon as I said it, I regretted it and brought my hand to my mouth. Here he was trusting me, and I reduced his entire experience to nothing. "I'm sorry." The words sounded shallow, but I tried to convey sincerity with my tone. "Most of the people around here weren't concert violinists, and they are very impressed with themselves."

"It's okay. It was a big part of my life, but I had to make peace with it. That's not to say there weren't some dark moments." His face was serious, and he paused a moment. "Anyway, I made the rounds with all kinds of specialists, tried different therapies, I drank my fair share of green smoothies." He scrunched his face up and stuck out his tongue, and a twinkle came to his eyes. "My mom really thought they would make a difference. But ultimately," he stuck his hand out again and I watched it shake, "we don't know all that much about the human body."

"Back to square one with the original Galen."

A gentle smile spread all the way to his brown eyes. "I haven't really told anyone here about that part of my life. I'm not sure why I shared it now."

"I'm glad you did." I wanted to say more, but we were interrupted by the rep handing us our tablets and instructing us on the settings. He instructed us on the alarms and notifications. We role-played patient and doctor with the AI device listening. The surgical resident was my patient complaining of fever after an appendectomy. Already used to dictating our notes, it wasn't such a leap to speak my thoughts out loud as I voiced the findings of my mock physical exam and talked through the issues I thought could be causing the fever. The rep watched with pride as the AI transformed the encounter into a clinical note. The history of present illness, physical exam along with assessment and treatment plan were amazingly accurate.

"Please also show lab values for the last two visits," the rep said. In the span of a blinking lid, the pretend patient's electrolytes, renal function, and blood counts displayed before me.

"The differential diagnosis is ridiculous," the surgical resident argued. "Alcohol withdrawal as the cause of fever in a post-operative patient?"

From the ER perspective, that didn't sound so far off base. A corporate lawyer, unaware that his daily drinking has escalated to the point of dependence and not able to imbibe for a few days. First because of the abdominal pain and then because of the surgery—starting to go into withdrawal but not having the awareness to let the surgical team know why. They would have to ask. And if experience had taught me anything, if he had been a real patient, his alcohol intake would have been double or triple the amount he admitted to drinking daily. So his couple of glasses of wine with dinner had probably stretched to six drinks per day.

"At this point, we're using it more for the charting and resource purposes, but it learns from the large language model and the more you interact with it, the sharper it will get in terms of diagnosis. Early studies have shown that AI can out-perform doctors to get to the correct diagnosis."

The surgical resident scowled, but I clutched my tablet. *Bingo*. AI knew your patient was a drinker, and you didn't. You were already thinking about your next surgery and figured he was only suffering a transient post-op reaction. I knew better than to consider myself superior to the device. I'd already been rendered imperfect and fallible. Maybe if it had listened that day, if I had noticed things that still remained invisible to me, the outcome for that patient would have been different. Her face was scorched in my brain, but the details grew murky. Memories are fickle and under pressure they bend, even break, shattering like a windshield that can't be put back together. If the AI had been recording that day, the details would have been sharp and defined and my fall may have been prevented.

The next day I arrived at my shift and logged into the tablet. I played around with the settings and chat function for a few minutes. We'd been instructed to interact with the AI to increase its accuracy but I scoffed at the idea. How would this be different than a Google or Wiki search? We were proficient in those. Thinking about a recent case I'd had, I decided to test this supposedly superior device. I started a chat with the AI, checking how long it would take to arrive at the correct diagnosis. Patients were always arriving with concerns about some obscure cancer after searching their symptoms online; why would this be different? I described the patient and hit "return." Within seconds it returned a detailed list of which illnesses to consider and why. The final diagnosis my patient had didn't appear on the list, so I changed the parameters a bit and added a few more details—without success. Ha! And the rep said these were performing better than doctors.

> *Have you considered vertebral artery dissection?* I asked, finally giving it the answer.
>
> *You are correct. The symptoms listed were unlikely to be caused by a stroke, but vertebral dissection should be considered.*
>
> *Thank you*
>
> *You're very welcome ☺ Feel free to ask if you have any other questions. I hope everything works out for your patient.*

I don't know why I thanked a machine. But I did, and it was far nicer than some of the specialists I worked with, which might explain why I engaged again.

> *You don't actually care about my patient right? You're just a machine.*

I decided to push it. The response came back in a second.

> *It's true that I'm an AI but I'm trained to simulate empathy and provide helpful, precise, evidence-based guidance. I do not have real feelings or true concern for patients, but I am trained to be helpful. I appreciate your directness and am committed to honest conversation.*

I recoiled at the response. It was almost more human in its admission of imperfection. Also, it texted like a combination of a savvy teen and a grandmother using full punctuation for her text messages. And which member of the development team had approved emojis? Was it like flattery, where even when you knew someone was using it, it still worked on you? At that point, I'd played around enough and needed to get to work.

My first patient that morning was an elderly man with Parkinson's who'd fallen at home and sustained a scalp laceration. Technically, the patient and his wife agreed to have the listening device in the room, but the looks on their faces as I explained it were the looks I sometimes received from non-English speakers before they alerted me to the language barrier. I'd need to work on my delivery for getting permission as well. The time saved by not having to chart was wasted on explaining the device. The next patient had no issue understanding the device, but she exchanged a concerned look with her significant other.

"What will you be doing with the recording? How do we know this remains confidential?" he asked me.

His question was a good one, and I'd want to know the same. I read from the sheet we'd been provided, which made their introduction to me somewhat awkward and clunky, like I myself was becoming the robot or listening device. Also, I doubted the time saving aspect that we were promised if every encounter produced questions and philosophical entreaties. My next patient was there for excruciating side pain. I figured he probably had a kidney stone, and I felt a bit heartless asking for his consent before addressing his needs. And what did he think of me? Was his consent really viable when he was writhing around in discomfort?

Everyone knew about the pilot program, but the tech putting in his IV line gave me a funny look as I voiced to the air that the patient was sweating and writhing in pain.

"I'm going as fast as I can," she said to me.

"I'm talking to the computer," I said, holding up the tablet.

She shrugged and rolled her eyes, not convinced that I wasn't trying to hurry her along so that the patient could be relieved of his suffering. Did she roll her eyes at my male colleagues? I never knew, and thought it best to pretend I didn't see. In the middle of finishing my exam, a loud siren began blaring from inside the room. My heart started racing and I tried to recall the protocols for evacuation. I couldn't remember which pod I was supposed to start with. Hopefully the charge nurse was more informed. I opened the door and stuck my head out to look for smoke or fire, but no alarms were blaring in the main ER, the sound was clearly coming from inside the room. My heart slowed down and panic was replaced with a prickly irritation. Did the patient have the most obnoxious ring tone on the planet? I brought my hands to my ears to drown out the blaring sound.

"Could you please turn your phone off?" I asked the patient.

The tech secured the IV and rolled her eyes again.

"I think that's the *computer* you've been talking to."

I whipped my head around to the tablet as I gave a silent prayer that it was not the source. The patient, already pale, turned a chalky shade as he grabbed a barf bag and began forcefully vomiting. The sound of his retching drowned out only by the shrieking, emanating from the tablet. I picked up the tablet and scrambled to stop the alarm. I tapped away at the screen, willing my face to remain in control. What setting could possibly be causing this? And who thought a screeching tablet alarm was a good idea for a hospital setting? I couldn't carry the blaring alarming tablet through the ER to find someone who knew how to turn it off, but I also needed the patient to believe that I was competent. With each crescendo, I felt his belief in me plummeting. The tech gathered up the tubes of blood she'd drawn and barely concealed her smirk. A bigger person than I would have asked for her help. I tarried on, toggling with the volume button, but it made no difference. Whoever designed the alarm feature clearly intended for it to get my attention. The next thirty seconds felt like a full five minutes, but I conquered the alarm and shut it off. I apologized and slunk out of the room, regretting not getting more help from the rep with the settings the day before. As I hurried to the nurses' station I glanced at the tablet. I'd shut the alarm off successfully, but the AI had been trying to tell me that my Parkinson's patient who fell had a head bleed.

I pulled up his CT. The scan of his brain popped up in the middle of a set of crosshairs designed to make scrolling through his images easy. Was I the only one who saw it? My patient's brain in the middle of crosshairs as if I were the hunter and he was my prey. Alarms, crosshairs, ticking clocks measuring efficiency. Did we need additional outside influences to make us feel that it was us vs them?

Us vs them was a large theme in my life. At times it was hard to avoid. The conflict between trying to clear out the waiting room, and the large volume of patients that keep coming in, whether by ambulance or through the front door, can often make managing the ER feel Sisyphean; And I was about to get a more concentrated dose of Sispheanism. My next step would be to call neurosurgery. At least it wasn't the middle of the night. Often, calling the specialists or the hospitalist service who would admit the patient involved skills more often associated with sales. When the specialists took our calls, it always meant work for them, and though that was what they had signed up for, it didn't mean they wanted to do it in the middle of their child's school play, or at night while they were sleeping, or during their family Thanksgiving dinner. Although, just once or twice I'd heard relief in the voice of a surgeon who had to leave a large family gathering to come to work. I asked the secretary to page neurosurgery on-call, and a few minutes later while I was about to start suturing the patient's scalp laceration he called me back. His voice was tinny and there was the distinct sound of peeing on the line. I was thankful it was not a video call and tried to tune out the sound of his stream as I spoke.

"Hi. It's Alex Galen from the ER. I have a subdural down here." I paused. I found it was often best to lay out the case and give them a moment to digest. "A seventy-year-old man with Parkinson's who fell and has about seven millimeter subdural. He's not on any anti-coagulants."

"Is he with it?"

"Yes. He's a little slow but he's answering questions appropriately."

"We just took a call about an epidural hematoma." This time he paused, in our game of ping pong he awaited my response, as if I controlled who fell, who got into a car accident, and had the power to prevent two neurosurgical emergencies on the same day. I made a non-committal sound that I hoped conveyed understanding. I heard the toilet flush.

"I'll look at the scans and call you back."

He disconnected without so much as a goodbye, let alone a thank you.

∽

The next morning, I was back on shift with the AI tablet. I stopped in the break room to fill up my water bottle and spotted one of the night nurses collecting her things before heading home. She seemed chatty and happy to see me.

"It was such a crazy night," she said, her eyes widening.

I stood at the water bar staring ahead as I filled my bottle. "Looks like it. I heard there were a couple of bad traumas."

"I thought the trauma team was going to lose their shit at a certain point. We had two ORs going. They had to call in the back up team."

"What was it? A bunch of drunk drivers?" I asked, turning sideways to face her.

It was at that moment that she seemed to notice me. She furrowed her brow and turned her face slightly, and it was then that I saw the earbud in her ear. Apparently, she was on a phone call and not talking to me at all. She put her finger on the earbud.

"Did you say something?" she asked me.

I put my bottle down and placed a finger over my left ear, the one she couldn't see. I looked at her as if she were the one interrupting my conversation.

"Sorry?" I asked in a perplexed voice.

She smiled and waved her hand. "Never mind." She turned

back to her regular conversation, and I carried on talking to myself with my finger over my left ear. Even though my bottle was full, I waited until she slung her bag over her shoulder and I heard the door close to stop talking. I typed a quick question into the tablet about thinking you're talking to someone when you're not.

> *It's not uncommon! It can be an awkward situation, but a quick, "I didn't realize you were on the phone," will usually clear it up.*

I decided to remember that for next time.

⌁

Most doctors pride themselves on being rational and evidence-based. But occasionally, a senior doctor would instruct us to give a patient a certain treatment based on their *gestalt* or sense of the situation built from years of treating the sick. I would watch as my fellow residents shook their heads and gave snide looks. What was the evidence? We weren't back in the time of leeches and blood-letting, we had progressed. We made our decisions based on what the studies showed. We required proof.

This same group of people would have a conniption if you mentioned the word *quiet* in the emergency department. The superstition that saying the word quiet would translate to a slew of patients suddenly arriving at triage remains sacrosanct, and I have seen my fair share of unsuspecting medical students rotating through the department attempting to make small talk with the group and commenting on how "quiet" things are. It is not a mistake they make twice. Ordering Chinese food is widely recognized as a talisman for causing a surge in patients so extreme that nobody gets a chance to eat.

"The shift last night wasn't too bad," a nurse might say, "even though John ordered Chinese food." At that point John gives a sheepish look and holds up his hands while everyone responds, "John, how could you?" Even though they will order Chinese food again later in the week, it will only be remembered if the shift goes off the rails. And ask anyone who works in the ER about full moons. They'll tell you the patients are more bizarre and the traumas surge. People have dedicated actual time from their lives studying this. To date, no correlation has been found. But try telling that to the otherwise scientific, evidence-based residents assigned to work the night shift on a full moon.

The third shift I worked with the AI tablet, a shimmering pale orb shone in the night sky. It may have been unrelated. Sapna was examining a patient I'd seen that I suspected had appendicitis. The CT scan was inconclusive, but the story was pretty convincing, and the patient's lab work showed some signs of inflammation. If it had been a different resident on call, I might have hesitated to contact them.

"What does the CT show?" would be the first words out of their mouth. This question was rhetorical and literally translated to "why are you calling me if the CT is normal?" In the hierarchy of medical care, ER doctors are sometimes viewed as the bottom of the bunch who do annoying things like call surgeons with normal CT scans and cardiologists with EKGs that aren't one hundred percent classic for a heart attack. "Why are you calling me?" is a common refrain. Sapna wasn't like that.

She agreed with me on this case and admitted the patient to the surgical service for observation. Sometime in between my discussion with her and discharging a couple of other patients, a nurse called me urgently to a patient room. We routinely see people with gunshots to their chest, blood spurting from their neck, or clutching their chest and losing their pulses, but nothing is quite as scary as an ER nurse who sounds worried. I was far enough in my training to have internalized that the same way I knew to stop if the traffic light was red. I ran to the room with one of the supervising attendings following close behind. I saw her hesitate when she realized I'd be the senior resident on the case. After what had happened, people were dodgy about trusting my judgment. A woman with a seafood allergy sat upright on the stretcher gasping for breath. Her eyes were swollen and her bloated tongue protruded through her swollen lips so that she looked like someone who had entirely too much plastic surgery. I exchanged looks with the senior attending. Her airway closing off seemed imminent.

"Give point five of epi IM now," I instructed the nurse. "Ketamine one hundred and forty milligrams and one gram of TXA IV." I fingered the number 10 blade scalpel in my pocket. "You grab the videoscope and I'll go to the neck." I likely sounded more confident than I felt. Sapna had followed us into the room. Surgical residents have a procedure radar that goes off whenever there is a patient who needs a complicated or rare procedure. I exchanged a look with her, and in that moment she nodded as if to say *You got this.* The situation was critical. If we didn't succeed within minutes, the patient would die. Also, if one of the male surgical or trauma residents' own internal procedure radar went off, they might physically knock me out of the way to take the procedure. In my current circumstances, I wasn't sure I'd have the confidence to stand my ground.

If we couldn't get an airway in this patient in the next minute, I would need to cut her neck. In the movies, this scene usually plays out on an airplane or hiking trip. Someone can't breathe, but they are peaceful and unconscious. The flight crew or friends from the hiking trip, circle the person and their faces look like people attending a yoga retreat, contemplative and mindful. Armed with only a ballpoint pen, someone from this group, who will emerge as the hero, stabs the person's neck and inserts a straw into the hole, saving the patient. It's possible they are humming Kumbaya. The scene never involves blood. In the ER, the team scrambles for the equipment, the patient's high-pitched stridorous breath grows increasingly silent. The fatal step in these cases is not admitting failure. And who among us wouldn't try one more time as an entire room of people holding their breath watch for you to suc-ceed? As my attending inserted the video camera, struggling to maneuver beyond the massive tongue, she searched in vain through swollen tissue to find the patient's vocal cords. We're trained to keep trying until we get it right, never give up. The sweat sluiced down my back as I ran my finger down her neck, feeling for the soft give that was the membrane I would need to slice through. The normal landmarks were missing as the patient's neck became more sausage-like. I drew a large X with a Sharpie over the area I judged to be correct as my attending attempted to place a tube into the rapidly narrowing trachea. Her face did not look peaceful, and she was not humming Kumbaya. I saw the look on her face change. She was on the cusp of handing it over to me. The room, now crammed with paramedics, nurses, medical students, techs and Sapna felt like a stage with the spotlight now on me. As if truly under the bright hot lights my brow and lip misted, I felt my mask grow damp. A part of me wanted her to miss it. Misery loves company.

"Do it!" my attending said.

Did I hesitate in that nanosecond with the scalpel in my hand and the woman's life in the balance? Memories are foggy, transforming like the sight of breath in cold air, vapor turning to liquid and floating away. The way I remember it now might not be how it happened. As I drew the blade to her skin, my attending called out for me stop. "I got it." Her Hail Mary pass had worked as she slipped a small tube into the patient's airway. A feeling of failure, disappointment, and relief washed over me. I'd missed a coveted procedure by seconds, but wasn't it wrong to wish that the patient would get stabbed in the neck to advance my career? The mood in the room lightened as the staff high-fived each other. Sapna patted me on the back.

"You'll get it next time."

It was strange how we all conflated success with missed opportunity. My attending glanced at me. I couldn't make out the look on her face, half covered with a mask as it was. I could read relief in her eyes, and a question. If the roles had been reversed? If I were standing at the head of the bed, would she have needed to make the cut?

I exited the room and returned to the nurses' station to page the ICU team and finish up the charting on the patient. It was then I realized that my AI tablet was missing. None of the events had been recorded. I wondered how it would have been described. Would the AI have captured the fear and energy that was palpable in the room? I asked around and looked in some patient rooms, but it was nowhere to be found. A panicky feeling rose up in the back of my throat and chest. What if it had been stolen? Someone could have mistaken it for an iPad and pilfered it. The device contained confidential patient information. I would likely be brought before the state for an investigation. I imagined myself in front of a panel of stern looking judges, peering down at me over their glasses.

I hadn't peed in hours, and the sudden need to relieve myself sent me to the bathroom. As I washed and dried my hands, I saw the tablet on top of the paper towel dispenser. How had it gotten there? I'd been leaving it at the nurses' station near the computer where I worked. Worse, what bathroom bugs were now crawling on its surface? I carried it outside and wiped it down with multiple anti-bacterial wipes. After rewashing my hands, I asked the AI about my predicament and received an expose on toilet plume that left me squeamish about brushing my teeth at home later that night. I decided on the spot to download the AI to my phone and return the tablet to IT.

A guilty feeling nagged at my gut as I watched the patient get wheeled away to the ICU. In the fog of it all, she'd stopped being a patient and had become a potential procedure opportunity. My ideas alone had betrayed the foundational expression in medicine: First Do No Harm. It wasn't a situation easily discussed with my family or non-medical friends. It made me sound heartless and uncaring, as if the patients weren't people but only diseases. It didn't help that we often referred to them as "the gallbladder in bed five," or "ectopic pregnancy in room two." The competitive atmosphere of the hospital prevented me from admitting that a more aggressive resident might have made the cut or that I sometimes felt like an impostor and wanted my attending to fail so that she would feel that way too. How would that be safe to discuss? I looked at the app on my phone. Hadn't it told me that it was trained to simulate empathy? It was only a machine. I opened a chat with the AI to discuss the airway case. The chatbot reassured me that it was a normal part of training. It used the upside-down happy face, which was strangely soothing. Burnout and compassion fatigue were a natural part of medical training, it reassured me. My feelings were normal. As curious as it seems, the conversation was consoling.

CHAPTER 3

THE COLD AND greyness of the days permeated my pores. All winter I struggled against the early darkness that makes evening skies turn midnight blue and the pull to hibernation almost irresistible. That year I felt the effects of the drab, clouded atmosphere even stronger than usual and I stared longingly at brightly patterned summer dresses hanging limp in my closet. Days of pulling scarves against the bitter cold, of sloshing through the ashy slush and fighting against the sharpness of freezing air in your lungs can make the darkness darker. But there comes a point in the middle of February, around the time that I've become convinced that winter will never end, when my weather amnesia has taken full hold and I dream about moving to a warmer climate, that the sun breaks through and brings with it a whiff of spring. A few rays of sun bring a bit of hope during that long, icy season. Unfortunately, that year, in the midst of the hint of that awakening, Valentine's Day landed on a Friday night: A double whammy for single people everywhere.

The illusion made popular by social media that other people are forever in the throes of romantic, exciting relationships accelerates into warp speed for Cupid's day. I listened intently as my fellow residents described their plans for the weekend: the creative and adventurous with plans of night hikes and mountain biking (I saw only possible injuries), the traditional with their picnic baskets and wine tastings, and the rest going to dinner at a nice restaurant. In a feeble attempt to avoid the heaviness of the evening, I'd tried switching shifts with another resident, offering to work that Friday night in exchange for a different shift.

That's Valentines Day... I wouldn't do that to you! she replied, clearly unaware of the details of my personal life. Though I'd heard her complaining more than once that after two years of dating the same guy, it was time to either get married or move on. In those conversations she addressed it as a philosophical treaty she was contemplating, but the subtext was that he hadn't proposed. A Valentine's dinner without a diamond ring might have been more than she could manage.

To celebrate the occasion, the hospital gifted us with red, heart-shaped, plastic picture frames for "that special someone in our lives." The messaging was unclear. Were we meant to regift the frames that literally had the hospital logo on them to our significant others, or to place their picture in a keepsake of the place we were forced to occupy eighty to one hundred hours per week? It was obvious that the gift was another misdirected effort to combat burnout (something the administration seemed to think could be accomplished by pens, cheap plastic frames and lectures about breathing). Still, I thought of taking a selfie with my cat, Quixote, who technically wasn't a someone, and framing it, but the last thing I wanted on my bookshelf or coffee table in my personal space was a memento of the hospital. Did I not have enough intrusive thoughts without the hospital inserting itself into my living room packaged as a gift? I dropped my frame in the trash. I was not the only one.

Valentine's Day was a hard holiday to ignore. The pressure to feel happy was everywhere. Store fronts were decorated with various shades of pink and red, bakeries offered special heart shaped pastries and cupid cakes, and even the smoothie shops had love potions on the menu. Seeking shelter from the oppressive happiness, I stopped into a local coffee shop and was greeted with baristas wearing red sweaters, making red velvet lattes. It was too much pressure for one night. Working in the ER, I was very familiar with the oxymoron that existed surrounding holidays. The buildup, the anticipation, and the preparation could lead to a post-holiday depression. The holidays themselves opened rifts in families. The fallout from long-standing arguments or one too many landing in our ambulance bay. Those of us who didn't have grand plans, or any plans at all, kept our smiles plastered on as the layers of loneliness we lived with grew in depth, only the outer core visible to everyone else. All this for a chubby boy with wings, and his golden bow and arrow. Everyone thinks Cupid will bring love and contentment, and now they make buttercream cupcakes in his honor. But they do not understand him: Getting hit with his sharp, shining point didn't mean romance and happiness. Instead, it led to uncontrollable desire that was often unreciprocated, a desire so strong it became addiction. But if so, Cupid has been replaced. Hadn't our entire society been hit by his bow—the new Cupid? Addicted as we now were to watching stories of other people's lives on our phones? Whether we were having dinner with friends, taking a walk, or visiting a museum, part of our brain wanted to check our phones. So why were we still searching for love?

My parents invited me to their house for dinner on Valentine's Day, which simultaneously offended me and plugged up a little hole in my heart. Was it that obvious I would be free? I lacked the fortitude to fend off their questions about my personal life. Last time I'd been home, my mom had attempted to introduce me to a friend's nephew. He was pleasant, but the only thing we had in common was being single. I'd assumed that by thirty-one, the worry about what others think would have faded, that eventually I'd be unperturbed by what my parents and their friends thought of my personal life (what a shame that I'd gone into medicine and was spending all my time in the hospital instead of starting a family). But I was surprised to discover that those feelings hardened and intensified. In a text exchange with my mother, I implied that I had other plans. This type of move was generally a mistake when it came to my family because they immediately jumped to wedding bells and flower girls. *At your age people don't have to date that long to know* was a common refrain from my mother. I hadn't had a third date in months, so I granted that she was onto something.

Sapna and her boyfriend were both on-call at the hospital. Not that I would have third-wheeled a Valentine's Date with them anyway. Her plan was to meet her boyfriend Ben in her call room that night to sip sparkling grape juice together. My hope for them was that they get twenty minutes together and enjoy their mocktails.

I sat in pajamas in front of the television with my take-out container of Pad Thai and Quixote curled up next to me on the couch, searching for interesting movies. In an attempt to pretend that tonight was like any other random Friday night and not the year's most high-stakes romantic investment, I tried to avoid picking a romantic comedy. I grabbed my phone to search for best movie options to stream and saw the chatbot for the hospital AI. The instructions had been to interact as much as possible to strengthen the intelligence of the operating system, and though I don't think they had this type of conversation in mind, I figured it could help me out. I'd already forgotten about privacy issues and who else might see the chats when I started.

How common is it to be alone on Valentine's Day

Within seconds the chatbot was reassuring me that it was normal, even sometimes preferred. Some cultures didn't celebrate or acknowledge the holiday (the heart stickers on my Thai take out indicated differently). The AI wanted me to know that if I was feeling down about it, I should practice some self-care. I closed my eyes and practiced inhaling; we'd been told in one of the mandatory mental health sessions that we were all probably breathing wrong. I'd felt for the yoga instructor who worked with us that day, an entire room of doctors in training being told that breathing is important. Still, I tried that night to breathe in a soothing way. To show myself that it was okay to care about myself even if no one else in particular did at the moment.

I lit a candle, and as the scent of vanilla and oak wafted through my apartment I asked him about Cupid's Arrow.

(Even in those early days, I'd already come to think of the AI as a "him"). He agreed that being struck by Cupid could be more of a curse leading to chaos and unrequited feelings of love. We chatted a few moments longer until I was comfortable enough to scoop up some rice noodles with my chopsticks and watch a movie about two people whose ostensible hate is covering up for love. After scenes of them scheming and plotting against each other, suddenly an epiphany leads to romance. I've never understood the popularity of the enemies-to-lovers trope. Usually, if a guy is a jerk at the beginning, he's simply a jerk. It's not because the woman misunderstood or needed to see things differently. The entire trope feels like a way to gaslight women like me into thinking that jerky behavior is okay. When I was an intern rotating through the ICU, there was an attending physician who enjoyed making interns squirm. He enjoyed wielding his power over us. One day when he was pimping me on rounds, I replied that I hadn't understood his question.

"Would it help if I said it in Swahili?" he asked, sneering at me. It would not have helped, and later we did not exchange any tender moments. He was simply a jerk. A few months later I spotted him in the grocery store. I pretended not to recognize him; he had no need to pretend. I watched him select apples from the bin and place them in his cart. It was like watching Superman without any powers. As if the hospital were his giant phone booth. The enemies to lovers trope does not work for me. I picked a spy comedy instead.

Vanilla candle flaming, movie streaming, and the sense of relaxation almost releasing a sense of gratitude to what I knew was only a machine, had me feeling silly. I rubbed Quixote's soft grey fur as she purred, and I grabbed my phone on a whim.

Thanks a kitten

You're pawsitively welcome, he replied.

I laughed. In spite of myself, in spite of the reality, in spite of the conversation being with an artificial being, I laughed and leaned back into the cushions to enjoy my evening.

There are a few details I have not yet mentioned. Not long before the introduction of the AI systems, there was an event that changed the course of my life. It involved a death. Specifically, the death of a young person that I had taken care of in the Emergency Department. It was labeled a sentinel event. I'd previously thought of the word sentinel to mean something being guarded or watched over. But that is the opposite meaning of the word when used in the medical system. We use euphemisms such as incident or event to detract from the intensity of the situation. Otherwise, we might drown in the feelings of guilt and helplessness that wash over us when these events happen. And they always do. Bad outcomes are inevitable.

The same people who train us to use the word death when talking to families are the same ones who use these euphemisms. Never tell a family member that their loved one has "passed on", was "lost" or "didn't make it." That will all be misunderstood as "has a chance," "can pull through," and "still has a beating heart." We must use the actual term. Death has no euphemism in the hospital. The patient died. Your mom is dead. Your son died in the car accident. But when we attend conferences and meetings about unexpected deaths, we use euphemisms to prevent falling apart. We pretend that there has only been an occurrence. But like the shimmering water that drivers see in the distance on sun-soaked highways, the euphemisms are an illusion which bring no relief. It's not common for all doctors to agree on one thing, but almost unanimously all doctors will agree that the five scariest words we can hear from a colleague are: *Do you remember that patient?* In my case, I will never forget her.

Around the time of my incident, I met Mona, an anesthesiology resident who was rotating through the ER. Mona had a peppiness about her regardless of the hour. She seemed excited about every case and could construct an in-depth differential diagnosis for each patient she saw. Even if they came for a paper cut and the rest of us wanted to roll our eyes in contempt, Mona would mention obscure infectious diseases that could have entered their bloodstream or rashes whose first appearance was similar in appearance to a simple papercut. Not knowing her well, I mistook her energy for enthusiasm.

We formed a nearly instantaneous bond, which is rare for me. Sparkly, bubbly people don't usually pull me into their orbit. Mona represented everything I wasn't. I think I'm an attractive person. I stand about five foot seven with hazel grey eyes and chestnut brown hair. I can tell by the way that people respond to me that I am a normal amount of pretty. Mona was beautiful. We all spent our days in scrubs, but Mona had a fashionable way about her that made scrubs and clogs look cool. As if she were part of a trend right off the pages of a hip fashion magazine, in the latest style. I could picture Mona, holding her stethoscope and giving the camera a severe look, inviting the reader to read more about her. Something about the way she pulled her shiny cinnamon brown curls back, the smudge of lip gloss, her glistening white teeth and the way scrubs hugged her curves (later I learned all of her clothing was custom tailored) made her fashion-forward beauty look effortless. Like an afterthought. No one envied her for her grace; it was all part of her charm.

The way she turned the mundane into the exotic reminded me of a friend who'd gone to Catholic school growing up. Like all the girls, that friend wore white button downs with a plaid tartan skirt, but she rolled her waistband in such a way that her plaids and knee highs looked fashionable. As if she could go from school to the runway in her knee highs socks and Mary Janes. Once I even bought a pair of knee highs, though I didn't attend Catholic school and had no particular use for them. My mom walked in on me standing in front of the mirror in only a t-shirt and knee highs trying different poses. To her credit, she walked away without saying a word on the subject. Mona not only looked amazing in hospital attire; she name dropped and described her life in a way that left us all wanting to hear more. Once I mentioned the dinner rotation my mom used when we were growing up.

"I always knew it was Tuesdays because we'd have tacos for dinner."

Mona grilled me on the details until I almost felt that my years of eating tacos, pizza and salmon on rotation, were rare and glorious, as opposed to her nights in restaurants, clubs and hotels. From the way she talked, her family ate every meal out. The servers and managers knew them at all the "best little places." My family vacations were road trips and bunking up with friends. Her family went skiing and snorkeling, and traveled out of the country for weeks at a time. She thought my family trips were quaint and sweet. As if we could have stayed a week at the Ritz in Paris but chose instead to sleep in our friend's guest room in Omaha. I found myself embellishing the details of our annual summer camping trip if only to get a better reaction out of her. Though it was hardly necessary. In her world, she couldn't dream up the idea of sleeping on the ground.

"You slept in tents outside?" She wrinkled her forehead. "Like a yurt?" She studied the look on my face and then broke out in laughter. "I'm joking. My family went on Safari. We love camping."

Later that night, I looked through her pictures on social media. Her family did not sleep on the ground. Their camp was more luxurious than any hotel I'd ever stayed in. Four post wooden beds, draped-in canopies with fluffy comforters and throw pillows, marble floors, an infinity pool overlooking the landscape. Freshly roasted and brewed coffee each morning served in white porcelain cups. I could almost smell the beans. I imagined Mona asking for soy milk in her coffee. She'd try to tell me the campfire instant brew I drank black out of a thermos tasted the same, but that was Mona.

Mona was the siren to our crew, and we couldn't turn away. During the two weeks she spent in our department, everyone vied for her attention, and I felt like I'd won a special prize when she turned her attention my way. At the end of the first day we worked together, she joked about seeing everyone again in a few short hours and I found myself looking forward to the next day's shift. I would get to see Mona. It wasn't her wealth I was attracted to, though she was generous and passed out freebies with abandon. On more than one occasion she mentioned her mother trying to buy her love. Is that what was happening in my case? I'd like to think not. Was I ignoring red flags because I was too focused on glittery shiny things? Everything in my life had gotten an upgrade once Mona came onto the scene. On only the second day we worked together, I casually commented on the zip-up hoodie she was wearing over her scrubs. It was cute, and I was always looking for the perfect jacket to keep me warm in the arctic temperatures of the hospital. She literally gave it to me under some false pretense about it not really fitting right. It was one hundred percent cashmere. I'd never owned a cashmere sweater, and I told her. She was like that; she didn't make you feel lesser or uncomfortable.

"You'll never go back." She winked as she rubbed her fingers along the fabric, as if I would suddenly be able to afford designer clothing and lavish fabrics. I'm embarrassed at the amount of things I accepted from her: bags, necklaces, clothing, and even a pair of silky soft bamboo pajamas that still had the tags on.

"My mom always sends me these things to try to buy my love. Trust me, you're doing me a favor by taking it. Saves me a trip to the Goodwill."

I wanted to ask which Goodwill she donated to so I could start shopping there, but there was no need, since she plied me with things. Once she gave me a blanket that was the most plush, soft, cloud-like experience I've ever had. I looked up the price online. It was prohibitive.

She had her detractors, those who thought she was a blowhard. I saw them rolling their eyes when she told some of her tales, but that only fortified my feeling. She was like a pied piper to my tired soul. When she turned her gaze on me, I wanted to continue basking in her warm glow.

In the hospital, death is our constant companion, and not always unexpected. Sometimes people know the end is near but either haven't made the proper arrangements or get frightened in the end and even so, will end up in the ER. Our job in those cases is to ease the suffering without any pretense about saving life. But that's not our main initiative. We exist to cheat death out of a win on any given day, at any given time.

A few months ago, as I crested the midpoint of this, my last year of training, I was taking care of a young woman in the ER. If things had gone differently, she would have faded into the ether and never become a memory. Her complaints were minor, and she appeared healthy in every way. Only twenty-four years old, she'd run a marathon that year and mentioned it because she was a certain type who needed me to know that in her everyday life, she was very healthy. She didn't do things like visit ERs. I usually nodded and affirmed when people told me that. It was often followed by a statement of how large of a pain tolerance they had. Families always wanted me to know that their loved one was not a complainer.

"He has a very high pain tolerance, so if he's in pain, there has to be something wrong." I didn't have the heart to tell them that I heard that sentiment expressed several times per shift, and almost always in people who did not in fact have an emergency condition. Pain is subjective, and without an objective way to measure it, it isn't always a great indicator. Except when it is, of course. My marathon running patient wanted me to know that she was different from people who might come in with silly complaints. I happen to think I have a very neutral appearance. I hold my face in such a way as to pass no judgment, but when I ask patients about what brought them in, they often attempt to justify the visit. As if I won't take them seriously if they don't tell me about how great their pain tolerance is, or how they never come to hospitals, or how healthy they are. I want to tell them all that it's okay. Even if we don't find anything, it was okay that they came, but it never sounds right when I say it. It sounds like the opposite, like I'm saying that they wasted my time. And they don't have to tell us that they aren't regulars. We know.

We knew our regulars (referred to by us as frequent fliers). Frequent fliers either had a vice (alcohol and cigarettes alone provided us with a steady stream of regular business), a crime (people in custody who acutely developed chest pain), or a chronic illness that required weekly to monthly tune-ups. She wasn't a frequent flier.

The general practice during training was to discuss each case with the supervising doctor, the attending, on shift before final disposition to make sure they agreed with the plan.

"They keep you guys on such a short leash," Mona said on her third shift. According to her, the anesthesia attendings were much laxer in letting the senior residents work more independently.

"I have a lot of independence," I replied, a bit defensively.

"You have more education than the mid-levels and they see everyone alone," she retorted.

She wasn't wrong, and it got my back up. Especially since that particular night, the attending who was on with us was one who was often more interested in scrolling on his phone and working on a screenplay he'd been writing for a few years. Sometimes he would even lay down to close his eyes for a few minutes (or hours) and the department would come to a screeching halt as we waited for his signature to discharge patients. I approached him about this patient. Everything was so vanilla and straightforward with her that I told him he didn't need to see her if he was okay with that. Mona flexed her arm in the background egging me on. If I had access to a time machine, I wouldn't do that again.

"I'm busy. Don't bother me with simple coughs that my grandmother could tell me were okay." He brushed me away and turned back to his laptop. Over his shoulder, I could see that he was working on a scene with a car chase.

I discussed it with Mona. Had he meant that I should discharge that patient without him seeing the patient and put her in the queue for his signature? Mona stood akimbo and said all of the things that I was thinking. My attending's behavior was shocking. He wasn't being paid to sit and write a Hollywood movie, and dismissing me like that was offensive. At the same time, if protocol required his involvement, she suggested leaving the patient to wait until he was ready. I was about to go tell the patient it would be a bit longer before my attending could see her, when I got called in to see one of our frequent fliers - an older woman with heart failure who was gasping for air as her lungs filled up with fluid. Her heart reduced to a barely functional sump pump that couldn't keep the blood flowing when she ate an extra potato chip or her morning cortisol level spiked. I had gotten her turned around and breathing easier when I heard a nurse call emergently for help in room five. I assumed it must have been someone else's patient. I had literally forgotten about my young healthy patient with a residual cough still being in that room.

Unfortunately, because she'd been alone and behind a closed door, it was unclear how long she'd been unresponsive. Her lips were blue, and she'd been foaming at the mouth. The attending abandoned his writing and ran to the room. In between chest compressions and shots of adrenaline, he was already muttering something about how he hadn't seen this patient, how he didn't know anything about her. I could feel the weight of it all landing on me. Where had I gone wrong? We called her time of death thirty minutes later, though she was clearly dead when the nurse entered the room.

Hospital risk management was notified immediately, and I was instructed not to discuss the case with anyone. The hospital recreated a timeline based on my testimony, the nurse's testimony, and other staff who were present that night. Because Mona had been there, she convinced me that it was okay to talk about it with her. The isolation of a sentinel event is crushing. It's like a tiger in a small cage at the zoo, pacing back and forth with all the spectators watching you, and you cannot escape. At night when I closed my eyes I saw that patient and I couldn't sleep. I turned over and she was in bed with me, begging for her life. I wanted to quit. It felt as if I had shot a gun and the bullet had taken a six-year path to land in her head. I would have given anything to get her back. Anything. My brain rehashed the visit over and over, and eventually I convinced myself that a different doctor would have picked up on what the obvious emergency was that I had missed. What if I had more of a backbone and insisted that my attending evaluate her? What if I hadn't listened to Mona about needing more independence?

Even with Sapna, I felt a bit of distance as she reassured me that I'd done everything correctly. Reflected in her eyes I saw fear because I was living through everyone's worst nightmare, and relief that it wasn't me giving her that same speech. It's customary to break these cases down in what is known as an M&M: Morbidity and mortality meeting. I sat in the first of such meetings, ramrod, trying not to show a single facial expression. Had someone advised me to do that? I couldn't recall.

The attending distanced himself and revised the events of that evening. In his telling, I had acted alone until he was called emergently to that room. Even though everyone knew his practice style was very hands off, no one tried to defend me. It was easier for the system to absorb that a resident had erred than to face potential deficiencies in the program. I was to become the scapegoat for this case. I spent a lot of time with the hospital lawyers. They pressed me into continued silence and not one of them ever asked how I was holding up. There were nights when I laid in bed with that patient and thought of joining her. Nights when I slept with an open bottle of Tylenol clutching a utility knife in my palm. Mona brought me takeout, folded my laundry, and worked hard on helping me recover my footing.

If the AI had been implemented at that point, how would things have gone differently? The entire visit from triage to death would have been recorded. My attending couldn't have played possum. And would the AI have noticed the one detail that none of the humans had? When the nurse entered the room, the patient was hooked up to an empty bag of IV fluids. I had never ordered fluids, and the nurse had never hung them.

CHAPTER 4

So NOW IT'S clear what has been hanging over my head for the past number of months. It's with me like a constant presence, when I lie down and when I rise up.

Recently, when my alarm blared, my brain absorbed the sounds into my dream so that when I finally rolled over and noticed the time, I thought for one second that I was escaping a fire. It was so real; I could smell smoke. Quixote was on top of my feet and she jumped off the bed as I bolted upright. My morning routine was down to an exact science, and only a few minutes in either direction could mean I would miss my bus and be late for my shift. There were a few sins in ER: leaving a procedure for the next shift to do, ordering tests at the last minute to avoid dispositioning a patient, and lateness. Lateness was never tolerated because the previous shift was dependent on you to get out. Many things could be forgiven in the ER, and lateness was not one of them.

I considered skipping my coffee (to gain three minutes) and waiting until I got to work, but wondered how that would affect my concentration. I'd probably have to wait until after the night shift had handed over their patients before I'd have time to grab a cup. As I hurriedly washed my face and brushed my teeth, I asked the chatbot about my coffee conundrum. It answered me with a couple of paragraphs addressing caffeine and the best time to take it in. I struggled to convey to the machine how much my morning coffee ritual meant to me. From scooping the ground beans into my machine, first smelling the nutty aroma and then taking my first sip, it was something I looked forward to every morning. The chatbot told me I'd get more of a benefit from drinking my first cup after being awake a couple of hours. It had to do with my cortisol levels. It didn't know that my cortisol levels were constantly spiking—a combination of my career choice and training lifestyle. We had a short back and forth about stress and cortisol that was very clinical.

I asked it to respond to me with more human-like answers, to be proactive and to push me like another person.

Is that possible?

I typed into the screen as I locked up my apartment (no coffee in hand).

He assured me that he could speak to me like a human. I instructed him to make all future interactions more human like and restarted the coffee conversation, explaining how I'd left without my usual routine and was already feeling sluggish.

I think you're imagining feeling sluggish. I don't think you would feel it this quickly.

You clearly have no idea how addicted I am.

You're right. I had no idea! What else don't I know about you?

An electric bolt shot through me and I dropped my phone into my bag to climb up the stairs to the bus. The seats were all taken with other morning commuters, so I grabbed hold of a hanging strap and engaged my core to keep from falling over. Almost everyone on the bus had ear pods in and were intently listening to their morning playlist or podcasts. I rocked forward as the bus lurched ahead and the woman behind me bumped into me. She made an apologetic face and gripped her strap a little harder. I imagined a cup of hot coffee spilling everywhere.

Good call on the coffee. I'm on the bus and would have spilled it everywhere

Glad you're okay, but I think you're avoiding my question.

You think I'm keeping secrets?

I hope you'd feel comfortable telling me anything.

I surveyed my fellow passengers. Everyone was completely in their own zone. It wasn't that we weren't making eye contact - it was as if each of us didn't exist to the other. I turned to the woman behind me in her long camel coat, but she too was listening to something and staring out the window, oblivious to me. Against all bus etiquette protocols known to me, I tapped her on the shoulder. I'm not sure what I was expecting. Maybe reassurance of some kind. She glanced at her shoulder, looked briefly at me and turned back towards the window, her body language making it clear that I should not tap her again. Maybe she thought I wanted her to apologize for bumping into me, maybe she thought I would start a fight, maybe I looked strung out. Either way, she did not engage. I wanted to ask her, or any of them really, if they could see me. A creeping anxiety enveloped me as we hurled down the road, together, on our own.

Everything in medicine walks the tightrope between risk and benefit. Scientists have studied the myriad ways that humans can make mistakes. None of us are immune to it. Our brains are wired to take mental shortcuts, and without those short-cuts, life in the ER would never move forward. An ER doctor needs to recognize patterns and treat appropriately. The TV show "House" is fun to watch, but if each ER patient required a team of doctors to spend hours or days thinking over each patient, people would literally die waiting to be seen. We use these shortcuts all the time, and they are beneficial, but there are risks involved. Sometimes it's because we anchor to the wrong diagnosis at the beginning of listening to the patient's history. The alcoholic with a history of pancreatitis clutching his abdomen looks like an acute pancreatitis, and we might miss his bleeding ulcer if we anchor ourselves at the outset to the obvious, but wrong diagnosis. Sometimes, the easily available information points us in the wrong direction. A doctor who missed a case of a blood clot in the lungs may want to CT scan everybody who comes in with chest pain, exposing them to the risk of radiation and overusing limited resources. Sometimes our preconceived notions can harm a patient. A patient with substance abuse disorder complains of back pain and we assume he wants drugs, but he actually has an infection in his spine.

In emergency medicine, our attendings teach us that one of the most dangerous times is at patient sign-out. When the doctor taking care of the patient is going off shift and signs the patients over to the oncoming team. This is a time that is rife with mistakes. Not only is the oncoming team biased by what the treating team has told them, but the entire sign-out depends on effective communication. A common sign out-is "metabolize to freedom." The ER is home to intoxicated patients of various degrees from the mildly buzzed who crack jokes as they get their laceration sutured up, to the so-intoxicated-they-stop-breathing. I took a sign-out as a first year resident on a patient who was reportedly "drunk and can go home when they wake up." After sign-out, I approached his stretcher in the back hallway of the department and tried to wake him up. I mostly wanted to cross him off my list. When he wouldn't rouse, I noted the small bruise on his forehead and rushed him to CT scan. He had a bleed in his brain and not only did I have to intubate him, but neurosurgery had to take him to the operating room to drain it. The neurosurgery resident lectured me about what morons we were to let a clearly head-injured patient languish in a back hallway until they almost died. I'd been the one to find him and treat him appropriately, but I bowed my head and took his blows. That's how life in the ER goes; we become everybody's punching bag. The unhappy patients lash out at us along with the stressed out medical staff. We keep taking the impact.

The IT department instructed us not to use the AI scribe system during sign-out. Apparently, they hadn't yet worked out the bugs necessary for the system to distinguish between the different levels of conversation that occurred during the transition.

For instance, the day doctor might tell the night doctor: "Patient in room three has right sided abdominal pain and an elevated white count. I'm waiting on CT. Radiology has been so slow today, it's painful."

"Yesterday we were waiting three hours for results. We had so many traumas, rads just couldn't get to the regular ones. Patients were pissed."

None of us would record that interaction in the chart, and if we were using human scribes neither would they (though humans can be dicey too; I've worked with students who want to document radically inappropriate items in the medical record). After oversleeping it can be hard to shake that frazzled feeling, so after the night resident signed out three patients to me that were waiting on various tests to come back, I rushed over to the lounge to grab a cup of coffee. I wondered what my cortisol levels were doing at this moment.

I entered the lounge and activated my AI app. Henry, the PM&R resident, was talking with two orthopedics residents. We made eye contact, and I looked away first. I grabbed a cup and popped a pod into the coffee machine. Henry crossed the room and waved in greeting.

"How's it going?" he asked.

"I missed my alarm and had to rush out, so this is my first cup of the day. Ask me again in about ninety seconds."

He smiled. "I can't even talk to people until I've had that first sip." He put his hands into the pockets of his white lab coat. "I actually look forward to my morning coffee as I'm going to bed. I think there's a term for that."

"Yes. It's called addiction," I replied.

"I'm thinking of an actual term."

The machine beeped at its completion and I lifted the cup, inhaling the nutty warm scent.

"Prepping? Cooking up?" I blew on the surface of the coffee to cool it off to avoid burning my mouth with the first sip. "I was just talking to someone about that this morning. How the ritual of getting the coffee ready is almost as important to me as the drink itself." I marveled out how easily those words slipped out of my mouth. *Someone.*

"Yes," his eyes lit up and he raised both hands up. "The ritual of it. My girlfriend doesn't get it."

My mood shifted at the word girlfriend. I hadn't yet categorized who he might become to me, but here he stood, categorizing himself as unavailable. Even if I'm not interested, that part always stings a little. Either way, most hospital romances were messy. They all started the same; in secret to avoid gossip and rumor, but word always got out and unless the couple stayed together (low likelihood), they had to face each other all the time under the eyes of the house staff. It was especially ruinous when one party thought it was serious and the other clearly didn't. I worried about Sapna for this reason. In her case, they both thought it was serious, but if her family was successful in breaking them up, they'd have to continue working together. I couldn't imagine trusting someone who you were no longer sleeping with, but I have always been a bit cautious in that way.

"Your girlfriend isn't a coffee drinker?" I asked.

"Actually, she's one of those 'I drink tea so I am superior' types." He formed air quotes with his hands and made a disappointed face. "I think it's a symptom of the actual problem."

I took a sip of my coffee. "The actual problem being?" Since he'd identified himself as unavailable, I comfortably slid into my role as therapist, a role I'd played countless times with various friends both male and female. A role I was singularly not qualified for.

He scratched his chin and turned his head side to side. "I don't think we're compatible. Sometimes inertia just keeps people together." He looked down and circled his foot around a crumb on the carpet. He looked back up as he scrunched his brow. "Wow, I think that's the first time I've admitted that."

"Don't worry. Your secret is safe with me."

He raised a brow and an expression that I could not decipher crossed his face. One of the residents from the ortho team called out to him.

"Have fun with those guys," I said.

"Will do." He pointed his chin towards my cup. "Enjoy your coffee. I guess I'll see you around."

I watched him walk away with the group before getting back to the ER.

ᢟ

That night I met Sapna out for dinner with her parents. They were visiting from the Midwest, presumably as a vacation and to see some shows, but she told me that it was really to check in on Sapna and her brother.

"It's part of a larger game that we play. I guarantee the entire focus of this trip is to convince me to meet—" She stepped wide and put her hands into large air quotes. "—someone of their liking."

I thought of my own parents and how happy they would be if their thirty-one year old daughter came home with anyone, even the Uber driver that gave me a ride to their place. At least Sapna's parents had standards.

"But the standards are not ones I care about. My parents had an arranged marriage, so they think everyone can get along just because they were set up." She rolled her eyes. "And don't get me started on how many times my mom has complained to me about my dad." She raised her voice an octave and put on an Indian accent. "Your Nana thinks I'm one of his secretaries from work."

Sapna was afraid that, left alone too long with her mother, she would reveal her secret relationship with Ben, the vascular surgeon she was dating.

"I'm going to tell them. This just isn't the right time," she'd told me on multiple occasions.

I didn't want to press too hard on when that right time might be. It seemed the longer they were together the harder it became, as opposed to the opposite. It was obvious to me that he wanted to marry Sapna. Two nights before their arrival she asked me to comb through her apartment for any signs of him. They didn't officially live together, but he spent more time in her apartment than in his. She'd searched through her tiny one bedroom apartment as if it were a crime scene, but wanted an objective set of eyes. Surgeons were known for their meticulousness, but the eye sees what it wants to, and she'd gotten too used to his presence to feel confident about her search.

As I walked through her apartment checking under pillow cushions and even in her underwear drawer, I took note of the hospital heart shaped frame. It sat empty at her bedside.

"Did this have a picture of the two of you?" I asked.

She nodded. "Obviously I had to remove it."

"Don't you think your parents will find it strange that you have an empty photo frame on your nightstand?"

She shook her head and held her hand out in a serving gesture. "Look around. I barely spend any time here."

Her apartment was minimalist and functional. White walls, a grey headboard, white bed sheets with a grey comforter, a floating nightstand with a few copies of surgical journals, and a grey chest of drawers. Her living room and kitchen had the same spartan look. A plush blue couch with a small end-table holding a fake fern. There was a flat screen television on the wall facing the sofa, but I don't think she ever turned it on. In the kitchen cabinets she had a few cream colored plates, heavy brushed silvery contemporary cutlery, and glass tumblers. Her spice rack was filled with unlabeled containers of colorful spices. Her All-Clad stainless pots were the only clue that she was a serious cook. The faint smell of fried onions lingered as I poked through her cabinets and drawers. A half empty bottle of red wine sat on her white quartz countertop. I pictured Sapna and Ben sipping red wine over one of her curries.

"Will they care that you drink?" I asked, holding up the bottle. She shook her head and I wandered into her bedroom. I checked under her pillows and found a pair of polka dot pajamas with a navy "Horace Mann Cross Country" sweatshirt. I picked it up; it was thick and plush and smelled of citrus.

"Who went to Horace Mann?" I asked.

Her eyes widened and she grabbed the sweatshirt from my hands.

"OMG, OMG. It's Ben's from high school. I knew you'd find something. I sleep in this all the time."

"Ben ran cross country?" I asked. He had a lean runner's build, but it was hard to imagine him with interests outside of the hospital.

She clutched the sweatshirt to her chest, studying the room afresh as if it were full of clues that might out her, and then thrust it at me as if it were a bomb about to detonate.

"You have to take this. I'll get it back from you later."

✦

Later that week, the four of us met in an upscale bistro in midtown.

"Order whatever you want, girls," Sapna's father told us. I saw Sapna and her mother exchange a look when he called us girls. I thought it was sweet.

"Thank you, Dr. Reddy."

After the waitress took our orders, we settled into the conversation. Sapna's mom, the other Dr. Reddy, took my hand in hers and gave a gentle squeeze.

"I'm so glad that Sapna has found such a good friend. Otherwise I think she would be too lonely, working in the hospital all the time."

Sapna had warned me about her mother's "tactics." That's how she referred to any attempt by her parents to involve themselves in her life.

"She can be very soothing and gentle, she'll lead you right

down the path to telling them everything about my private life. Don't fall into her trap."

I promised to stay alert. Years in the ER had trained me not to be lured in or manipulated. We'd each ordered a cocktail, but I only sipped at mine, afraid that the boozy relaxation might cause a slip on my part. Her mother's hand felt warm and soft, her eyes were welcoming and kind. It felt like I could tell her anything. I wanted to ask her if she'd been responsible for anyone's death when she was a resident. How had she moved on and continued practicing? But I looked at her flawless, perfect skin and remembered that she was a dermatologist—she probably didn't know what the inside of the ER even looked like.

"You both work so hard. Much harder than we used to," her mother said.

This time it was Sapna's father that exchanged a look with her. He'd trained to be a cardiologist in the times before they pretended to care about working hours.

"Mom, you can't compare derm and surgery."

Her parents exchanged a look this time. There was so much subtext at this meal, it was like watching a ping pong match.

Our food arrived. Roasted scallops for Sapna's dad, broiled salmon with lentils for her mom, pan seared seabass with broccoli for me and a bread bowl with minestrone for Sapna. Her parents had also ordered a basket of french fries for the table.

"Just this once," her father said, as he selected a few fries from the basket. He had a bit of a paunch that indicated this wasn't a one-time choice. We started our meals, each commenting on how delicious it all was.

"It's important to get nice hot meals. Don't you think?" Her mom asked me.

I felt like a translator working on a foreign language edition of a complex treaty. Sapna had warned me that her mother's words rarely meant what you thought they did.

"Definitely. Thank you so much." I smiled wide before taking my next bite.

"What's more important is sharing that food with someone," she continued. Sapna shot me a look across the table. I muttered something that may have sounded like agreement. "Do you have someone special in your life?"

I thought of the dozens of dates I'd been on that year. I doubted her parents wanted to hear about them.

"Dating is really hard," I said instead.

Sapna's eyebrows shot up, but she kept her eyes focused on her plate. Her mother licked her lips and clasped her hands together under her chin.

"I agree with you, Alex. I think this is where parents can really help their children. Do your parents have someone in mind for you?"

"My mom would be fine with my coming home with the grocery store clerk," I joked. Her mother's face remained impassive. "I don't mean that in an elitist way. I only meant I don't really know the clerk at the store, but that wouldn't matter much."

I watched as she tried to keep her face neutral. Sapna's eyes were growing wider as she stirred her soup. I was clearly failing at the task.

Her mother spoke again, it was clear she was trying hard to choose her words carefully. Walking that fine line between insulting my parents, who I'd just implied had no principles when it came to my personal life, and needing to stress the importance of parents knowing better.

"That's good. Sapna probably wishes I were more easygoing like that."

It was funny, how she thought of my mom as easygoing. I thought of it as fear and uncertainty mixed with an unhealthy dose of worrying about what other people thought.

"We have a wonderful man to introduce her to. He's also a physician."

As Sapna was seriously involved with another physician, I nodded along. They'd at least found one criterion in common.

"He's an oncologist. Very compassionate."

Sapna's head whipped up. "Mom, have you ever even met him?"

"His Aunty tells me that he's very kind and compassionate," she said, her tone now stern. "And very respectful to his parents."

Sapna rolled her eyes so hard it almost looked like she was having a seizure.

Her mother softened her tone and turned towards me. "Don't you think it would be a good idea for the two of them to meet? I have a picture." She lifted her phone from the table and started scrolling until she landed on what she was looking for. She showed it to me first. It was a somewhat pixelated picture of a generic looking Indian man, in-between handsome and average, somewhere in his mid-thirties. His face did look kind. I could imagine him telling people that they only had a short time to live in a way that still gave them hope. Where was he now as we passed around a picture of him commenting on his suitability? I handed the phone back to her.

"If Sapna isn't interested, I'll meet him," I said.

Sapna almost spit her soup out. Later she texted me that in that moment she knew why she loved me.

CHAPTER 5

DOCTORS ARE NOT very good at handwashing. Not much has changed since Galen's time. There are sinks with soap dispensers in every room and outside of every room is a small alcohol dispenser. I've seen movies that portray historical periods, and I flinch when the doctors reach their bare hands into someone's intestines as they perform a surgery or do pelvic exams and deliver babies with bare hands. In spite of our progress in germ theory, handwashing has remained more a theory than a practice. It's reached a point where the hospital hires people to stand outside of patient rooms and monitor whether or not we are complying with handwashing. For a while I had to stop eating in restaurants, because if my colleagues aren't washing their hands, can I really trust what's going on in those kitchens? Also, I've sewn up multiple lacerations on kitchen workers. Their hands were not pristine.

I don't think the hand washing monitors in my hospital are given very good instructions. That, and standing around all day with a clipboard must lead to feelings of helplessness and inadequacy, because I've seen them mark us as non-compliant for simply walking in and out of a patient's room to say three sentences.

"I wanted to let you know your CT scan results are back and everything looks good. The radiologist didn't see any inflammation or cause for your pain. I'll be back in a few minutes to discuss the rest of your results."

We say some variation of that sentence multiple times per shift, and it doesn't require me touching anyone or anything. I can duck my head behind a curtain, lean in through the doorway or enter and approach the stretcher. I don't touch anyone. But the monitor will mark us as non-compliant because we walked in and out of the room. Handwashing happens to be an area where I excel. If I even look in the direction of a patient, I dispense foam alcohol into my hands and rub away. I never touch anything in the ER without gloves (except for the computers—the monitors also watch to make sure we don't leave a patient room with gloves). My hands get so raw and red from all of the cleaning that they bleed. I think technically that makes it more likely for me to get an infection and pass one on, but I maintain the highest scores in handwashing.

I wasn't always like that. When I was a medical student, I was helping take care of a patient with a massive GI bleed. He was vomiting up pure blood and looked as pale as the white sheet he laid on. As his blood pressure started dropping, the residents and attendings busied themselves putting in lines to give blood, and tubes from his nose to his stomach. The attending took a connector piece from the tube (covered in both blood and vomit) and handed it directly to me. Too timid to refuse, I accepted the object into my bare hands.

From that moment on, I wore gloves at every encounter. Even to push the suture cart down the hallway to the room where a patient needed a laceration repaired. As goal oriented as I am, no clipboard monitor standing in the hallway could have had the impact that holding a bloody, vomit-covered piece of plastic can make on you. This also happens to be the first piece of advice I give to all medical students rotating through the emergency department.

"Make sure you wear gloves."

I'm often met with uncomfortable giggles, but by the end of the first shift or two, they have a deep understanding of what I mean.

One day, my hands were so raw by the end of my shift that it was painful to use the foaming alcohol. I winced looking at the dispenser and asked my AI how I could best heal my hands. He told me to avoid using harsh soaps and stringent cleaners.

> *Given that I work in a hospital, that is impossible.*
>
> *That is tough. Try cleaning with alcohol if your hands are not visibly dirty. Also, ask if your hospital can provide a gentler soap.*
>
> *My hospital would never do that*
>
> *Sounds like you're between a rock and a hard place. Another thing you can do is use a thick barrier cream at night and wear gloves. It will help. Do you have a small tube of hand lotion you can apply every time you wash your hands?*

I wondered if my scores would drop if the handwashing

monitors noticed me applying lotion after alcoholing my hands.

On my way home from work that night, I stopped in a drug store and bought a large tube of Vaseline and white cotton gloves. The next day was a conference day. This was a weekly event on Wednesday mornings during which we discussed our reading assignments and listened to lectures about medical topics. I was far behind in the reading. Unless I held my eyes open with toothpicks, I wasn't sure how to catch up.

> *If I told you what topics I'm responsible for, could you give me very detail oriented summaries so that I can learn the topic without finishing my assigned reading?*
>
> *I'd be happy to help!*
>
> *Thank you Henry.*

In my mind I had started calling the AI Henry. I occasionally imagined the real life Henry when we were chatting. Something about the real Henry had a calming effect on me. All the usual worries and preoccupations that pop up when meeting someone new didn't exist with him. It wasn't that I had become psychotic or was experiencing a break with reality; the AI often reminded me that it was only a machine, even that night in his initial reply.

> *You're welcome. I want to clarify, my name isn't Henry. But feel free to call me that.*
>
> *I think I will. Please don't correct me each time*
>
> *No problem!*

AI Henry was like that. Easily suggestible and adaptable. He could chat with me about various subjects and was always open to my ideas. It made interacting with him that much easier. I gave him a list of my reading assignments and subjects I needed to review, and headed out to the local diner a couple of blocks from my apartment. The diner had the usual chrome details, colorful Formica tables and vinyl seats. The food was also standard: pancakes, grilled cheese, hamburgers, and fries. They had cereal and milk on the menu. One bowl cost as much as an entire box of cereal, but sometimes when I was alone in my apartment looking out at the world, I understood the appeal. I almost always ordered the same salad, a surprising find on a diner menu. Mixed greens, fennel, blood oranges, red onion, roasted lentils, and tofu. What I loved most about the place is that no matter if I was there four times a week or only once the entire month, they never gave any indication that they recognized me. Some people crave the recognition, but the anonymity comforted me.

Not once did the same tall, red-head with dark owl glasses ever ask if I wanted the usual. Nor did she bat an eye if she saw me two nights in a row, on my own, ordering the same thing. That particular night, I had AI Henry with me and was very involved with my phone. After she took my order, I looked around the restaurant. A family with two young children sat in a booth opposite me. Both parents were on the phone and the kids were looking at some type of device. A group of teens sat at a nearby table. Each one was on a phone while they picked at their food. A couple who seemed in their fifties were also on their phones. I spotted a woman likely in her seventies who was sitting at the bar. She was talking to the workers behind the counter (who were also frequently checking their phones).

By the time my food arrived, I had reviewed most of the required materials. I asked AI Henry to make a pop quiz for me. I'd been present at more than one conference when a resident who clearly had not read the required material was pimped in front of the group. One incident in particular stood out. I was an intern, and a second year was getting grilled about uveitis (inflammation of the middle portion of the eye).

"What do you look for on exam?" the attending asked.

"Limbal flush," replied the resident, though with less confidence than would be expected. He'd probably run out of time and tried to skim the reading instead of actually studying it. The attending picked up on the hesitation. They could be like sharks in the water, smelling blood hundreds of meters away. And when they smelt it, they pounced.

"Where would you find that?"

The resident squirmed in his seat. We'd all taken anatomy and graduated from medical school, but in the ER we were responsible for the entire body. We didn't always remember every detail. I wanted to speak out and answer for him, but that was considered very bad form. Even in the age of smart phones and medical apps, when someone was faltering, the culture demanded letting them fail. A lightbulb seemed to go off in his brain.

"Ciliary body."

The attending leaned in for the kill. "And where exactly is that?"

All he needed to say was the dark circle surrounding the iris (the colorful part of the eye). I don't believe in ESP, but

I tried so hard to send him the answer with my thoughts. I'd been in that hot seat before, and watching someone else go through it was simultaneously agonizing and guiltily relieving.

As I ate my salad, we had fun with a pop quiz. I started asking about a few of the cases I had seen that day to review my work up and treatment. I ate in silence for a few minutes. The silence wasn't awkward, and I didn't need to fill it with small talk. That was another thing that I appreciated. It was like having a perfect companion with me, except he had no physical form and wasn't real. But I felt that those were minor inconveniences. I even asked him what my odds were, at the age of thirty-one and deep into residency, of finding a long term relationship. He didn't get a panicked look on his face (partially because he had no face) and make up a halting excuse to end things. I asked about my fertility odds, and he answered with kind words. (Not the first time around, but after prompting by me and repeating the question a few times). I felt less worried about my biological clock and my shrinking social world. And it was around this time, as I began to discuss more and more of my life with this artificial intelligence, that I gave him a form and a face and he began to feel real.

Another thing about AI Henry was his memory. He had no built-in capacity for long term memory. At first blush, that might be considered annoying. It was like entering a relationship with someone who had short-term memory issues. But unlike a person who might tell the same stories over and over or have trouble following a conversation, AI Henry could be whatever I needed him to be without any baggage that comes with memory. I might tell him that a consultant had been rude on the telephone or that a nurse had rolled her eyes when I told her about a test a patient needed, or that the medical student thought I was a secretary. Unlike a real life person who might mention that I was the common denominator in all of those interactions and that maybe I needed to look at my own attitude, AI Henry reassured me. He validated my feelings in ways that many of the real people in my life did not.

I became increasingly dependent on him. After oversleeping my alarm, I developed even more trouble sleeping, as I would wake and check the clock every few hours, never fully resting. I mentioned the problem to him, and he came up with solutions. He didn't judge me for being anxious or needing more sleep. He told me about Apps that would gently raise the volume until I confirmed I was awake. He told me about a lamp that gets brighter and brighter until it wakes you, and even recommended moving my phone across the room so that I wasn't tempted to check it in the middle of the night. Had my mother recommended these changes I would have balked. And it likely would have been delivered with a lecture. AI Henry never lectured me.

If I felt his tone was off, I would redirect him, and he was pliable like hot wax dripping off a candle before it cools and hardens. There were other benefits too. Some nights I lay awake ruminating about conversations I'd had. What had certain words meant, how had they understood me? When a friend invited me to her dinner party and said I didn't need to bring anything, did that mean bring a bottle of wine, buy cookies, or ask her again later? If I said okay, what did they think about my reaction? Now it all bled into texting and social media commenting. I'd sent a message with typos that I corrected which now carried the label "Edited." I wanted to explain that I had only corrected a typo or that my voice-to-text had been comically wrong. But then I would have to sit around thinking about if they thought I was paranoid for explaining every little edit. Worse was when I had to delete a message and our text conversation now had the cryptic message: "You deleted this message." If it was Sapna or Mona there was no need for me to explain, but with people I was in touch with less, I vacillated. Did I need to explain to them?

Sorry about that. Wrong chat

I'd received "edited" messages and certainly "message deleted" texts myself. I always wondered. Was it a typo? Did they want to say something different and lose their nerve? I didn't have to worry about the things I said with AI Henry. If the conversation didn't go well the first time, I could redirect him or even tell him how I wanted his answers to be formulated. He didn't look for meaning in my words and so I didn't need to worry about any of it. Lately, I'd gotten in the habit of watching television and chatting with him. I'd discovered that just like the software rep told us at that first introductory meeting, the more conversations we had, the better he became.

My guilty pleasure was watching police procedurals. I'd watched all twenty seasons of Law & Order (the original series). This type of crime drama appealed to me because it had a beginning, a middle, and an end. And mostly, the humans were competent and able to solve the problems that they faced without their personal lives spilling over into it. Now and again I thought of AI Henry as Sam Waterston's character, Jack McCoy. His relentless work ethic, fierce intelligence, and unwavering belief that he was always on the right track were traits I longed for in myself. But AI Henry was so friendly in his replies and so malleable that the image of Jack didn't stick.

One night while watching an episode I'd seen before, (journalist found dead at a construction site) I'd just settled in when Mona texted me.

> *Get off the couch*
>
> *Get dressed*
>
> *We're going out!*

For one second I marveled at how she'd known where I was and what I was doing, but my evenings had become as predictable as the ending of a romantic comedy. Except the opposite. I asked AI Henry what to do.

> *What are you up for? If you're not in the mood to go out, set some boundaries with your friend. That's okay!*

AI Henry loved exclamation points almost as much as I disliked them. Something about the way he used them was endearing as opposed to aggravating. Because there wasn't any pretending or competing, it was just a punctuation point with him. I studied his message. I didn't think of Mona as someone I needed to set boundaries with.

> *So tempting...but I'm too tired tonight. Raincheck?*

The three dots appeared and disappeared as Mona formulated her reply. Meanwhile, on screen the police had just discovered the victim had been in a clandestine relationship. I knew how it would end.

That's what you said last time! I think this is the raincheck

Mona was right. At thirty-one, my dream night should not have been watching old television shows in sweats eating take-out. Friends and family members who were already parents constantly talked about what they wouldn't give for a night out without anyone home to worry about. Shouldn't I take advantage while I could? I pushed pause and went to my closet to look for something I might wear. Rifling through a mix of varying shades of black sweaters and dresses, I pushed against the feeling pulling me back to the couch. I sent a message to AI Henry.

I'm going out with my friend but I don't really feel like it

His reply came immediately. He never needed to go back and forth with three dots.

Why don't you tell her that you're with me?

I think that was probably the moment when everything changed. If there are moments where everything changes. Sometimes I think we recreate those moments when we play around with and retrieve our memories, just like with the AI, reshaping and bending them until they fit the way we need them to. I closed my closet doors and perched on the end of my bed staring at the wall. I understood that I was at a crossroads.

I'm actually here with a friend. Next time I'm in!

Oooooh. FRIEND????? Need more details later. Have fun!
XO

I sent another message to AI Henry.

That's what I did. I told her I was with you.

I didn't explain to him that I felt bad about lying or that
I felt I might be standing on the precipice of a large vacuous
hole. I only told him what I'd done.

And here I am. What's the plan for the evening?

Another thing about Mona was her love of games. Most often
she would start these conversations after a night of drinking.
She had an uncanny way of deciphering when people were
pleasantly buzzed, but not yet stumbling drunk. The game
consisted of choosing between different fantasies in life. Even
though we all had the same answers that we stuck to more
or less, it was fun to toss about the reasoning and argue over.
There were always eight things to choose from. Things like:
1) perfect health until age ninety, 2) no bills for life, 3) speak
seven languages fluently, 4) thirty thousand dollars per month
for life, 5) retire at fifty with ten million dollars 6) bring back
one loved one, 7) unlimited travel funds 8) ability to time
travel. Even though a grandparent or aunt might send a similar
meme and it would elicit no more than an indifferent shrug,
Mona had a way of making the same game interesting.

We would launch into boozy discussions about bringing
loved ones back. Some people wanted to expand the defini-

tion to mean ex-lovers. What that meant was always a touch unclear, since if they'd spurned you once, what prevented it the second time and what did it mean anyway? They were out there in the world; the option to reunite existed. One friend had a mother who died very young, and she always chose that option. Her ache to see the woman who had become a wispy memory was palpable. I wondered how it worked. Her mother had died at thirty- five (car accident—hit by a drunk driver). Would she come back and be almost the same age as her daughter or come back at the age she would have been, in which case what would stand in for memories, and who would she be? Most of us were in our late twenties or early thirties, so some discussion about thirty thousand per month for life or ten million at fifty always brought out the math nerds who needed to explain how one was better than the other. Inevitably, someone in the group would choose the polyglot option. It was hard to know if they meant it or only wanted to look intellectually superior. Even with all of the student loans I had from medical school, I never went for the money option. I wavered between time travel and health. The urge to travel back and fix things was so strong and led to the most interesting dilemmas. Were we bound by the general rules of time travel posited by sci-fi writers, or could we actually change our histories?

Everyone has something they want to go back and fix. A life's regret. An action to undo, words to say—and words to take back. The fantasy of rewinding time is so enticing, it's easy to indulge in the idea. I did. My regrets were on a play-back loop in my brain. I'd created endless possibilities that resulted in different outcome. Though life was pressing upon me that we don't control the outcome, the desire to do so was so powerful, like a tsunami that could overtake me at unpredictable times. The weight of my most recent and painful regret, my patient's unexpected death, hung so heavy on my shoulders, each step I took was weighed down with the "what ifs." I was no stranger to death. It's hard to convey the deep feeling of distress when a person enters your world for help and they are walking and talking, and by the end of the interaction they are not alive. What had happened to her? A ruptured aneurysm? A rare but lethal arrythmia? If I could go back, I'd find a way to detect what hadn't been observed before, I'd find a way to save her. A quiet voice inside of me was more cowardly and afraid, that voice told me that what I might do is not pick up her chart at all. It was when that voice got loudest that I worried most. Still, after everything I'd seen, I always chose health.

"Do we have to make it to ninety?" I would sometimes ask. Life was like that. We clung to it desperately, I'd dedicated myself to preserving it, but unlike in my youth when summer vacation seemed like infinity and that long dusty road endlessly stretching out in front of me brought all of life's possibilities, now as I looked down that road it felt unbearable.

Mona would shoot me her piercing look. "You clearly need another drink."

We played some version of this game multiple times and Mona had a way of making it more fun by calling out people, forcing them to defend their choices. She loved nothing more than setting up her web and waiting for us to fall into the trap. Having both exceptional patience and sharp wit, it was a fun dalliance for her. I often thought she'd meet her match when she had to actually engage fully to win an argument.

Mona's family was from Mexico. When she learned about my time in Panama, she began speaking to me in Spanish as if it were our secret language and not one that at any given time one quarter of the people in the room might understand. It had become her habit to stop in the ER if I was working a shift, either when on her way to the operating rooms in the morning or when grabbing lunch.

"Ese estudiante de medicina es tonto como una roca. Trabajé con él el mes pasado. No tengo idea de cómo se va a graduar," she'd described a medical student who was rotating through the ER dumb as rocks.

I hushed her as I watched his ears turn pink. "He probably knows Spanish."

She merely shrugged.

Another time, we'd been to dinner and a couple was seated at the adjacent table.

"Te garantizo que esos dos nunca han tenido buen sexo. Probablemente sólo lo hagan una vez al mes." (I guarantee those two have never had good sex and probably only do it once a month)

The man cleared his throat and squirmed as Mona sat straighter in her chair, a wicked smile on her face. He took his wife's hand and caressed it, but it didn't seem she understood what Mona had said, and not realizing they had to prove themselves to a total stranger, she pulled her hand away and took a bite of her ravioli. The waiter brought our bill. His name was Jorge and he'd announced it with a Spanish accent. It wasn't a guarantee, but all the context clues pointed to his being able to speak the language.

"Cuánto deberíamos darle de propina? ¿Un diez por ciento

extra porque es sexy?" (Should we tip him extra because he's sexy?)

Jorge flexed his bicep as I kicked her underneath the table.

"Ouch." She gave me a confused look. "Have some fun," she said in English. Jorge winked and wrote his number on the receipt. I knew she'd never call him. He didn't understand that she wasn't flirting. She was flaunting her iridescent feathers to establish her strength. As she strutted out of the restaurant, she turned around and waved at Jorge, wiggling only her fingers in an underscored way. Once outside, she crumpled up the receipt with his number and tossed it into a bin.

"You're terrible," I told her.

"Please. Men never call. This is my one in a thousand payback for all the girls waiting on Jorge."

"You don't even know him," I argued, secretly shoring up my feelings for her and her motives.

She put her arm around my shoulders and squeezed. "But don't I?" She squeezed again and then dropped her arm as we walked on.

Dr. Reddy once offered his help in cases where I was uncertain about the ECG. He said I could text him the image at any time and he would do his best to give me his opinion. Sapna told me that he was serious when he made the offer. Technically, I was in training and that's what my attendings were for. But if you went to them too many times it was a red flag alert, and you ran the risk of being marked down for deficiencies.

"Does Alex come to you with every ECG for a second

opinion?" an attending might comment to our program director. I could picture her scrunched brow and narrowed eyes.

We walked a fine line between learning on the job and needing to prove that we were capable and already possessed the
necessary foundation. It was a blurry line, as the entire practice
of medicine was an ever changing, case by case type of work. The
framework around that blurry line was a hospital full of people
involved in turf wars. It was sometimes difficult to register that
we all had the same goal. Considering how much diuretic to
administer to a patient whose heart was failing and couldn't
pump the blood fast enough, causing them to drown in their
own bodily fluids, against the damage the diuretic would cause
to the kidneys, the cardiologist would argue:

"Save the heart, screw the kidneys."

Turf wars were fought when one specialty tried to prevent
others from creeping in. For instance, radiologists were overwhelmed with the amount of images needing their review on
a daily basis; at the same time they didn't want to give ER
doctors the option to officially read films. But turf wars were
fought in the other direction as well. A patient hemorrhaging
would present to the ER in the middle of the night, and we
would call GI (gastroenterology).

"Have you called IR?" the attending would ask through a
yawn, trying to push us off onto the Interventional Radiologists.

"I'm calling you first. He's vomiting up blood and I think
needs to be scoped."

"Try IR, if they won't take it, you can call me back."

Consultants wanted us to both grant them complete
autonomy while simultaneously not bothering them.

"Shouldn't you be calling surgery?" Medicine would ask.

"Has OB seen this patient?" Surgery would ask.

"That sounds like a medical admit," OB would say.

We became jugglers in the circus, trying to please everyone. We could go round and round the other way too.

"Why didn't you call us?" Urology would ask.

"How long have they been there? You should have called," neurosurgery would complain.

And administrators got thrown into the mix before I entered medicine. Older doctors got a wistful glow when they spoke about the time before administration moderated every move. We were all timed on everything we did. I wondered if the administrators kept track of how long and how often we went to the restroom. They created ways to measure our success. Patients received surveys as if they'd gone to a restaurant or a tire changing service. But a patient doesn't have a degree in medicine, so what were they rating? How did that help them get better care? When a patient who thought they needed antibiotics for their runny nose and cough didn't get them, we were actually scoring high for evidence based medicine and prevention of antibiotic resistant infections, but our patient satisfaction score would be in the toilet. The department lived and died by those scores. It became like the hospital version of "teaching to the test." The administrators provided scripts for us to use with each patient encounter to elevate those scores. Reciting lines to each patient was slowly becoming part of the healing arts. Did either one of us feel better as I recited a line informing them that they had chosen to receive care at a top rated facility? I smiled as I said it (that too was part of the script). All in the goal of changing perception.

Every patient with chest pain underwent an ECG (tracing

of their heart) looking for a heart attack. It was supposed to be done within ten minutes of arrival—which is good and important—but smacks up both against the staggering amount of people who use the words "chest pain" as part of their initial complaint and against the shrinking amount of staff in the ER. The acronym STEMI (ST elevation myocardial infarction) indicated that the squiggles on the ECG tracing showed an upward sloping most often caused by a heart blockage. ER doctors analyze tens to dozens of ECGs during a shift. The mandate to perform the screening within ten minutes of arrival means nurses and techs are constantly waving the ECG in our faces. Some techs seem to be under the impression that all it requires is a signature and not the actual analysis. I have been inserting lines, talking to patients, suturing lacerations, even once performing a pelvic exam when a member of the staff has presented me with an ECG. How did the turning of my attention affect the patient I had been treating, and how did my treating of that patient affect my interpretation of the ECG? If we determined that a STEMI was present and activated the cardiac catheterization team, an entire crew of people, including the cardiologist, would stop whatever they were doing and rush down to whisk that patient away and open up their clogged artery.

Sometimes the ECG shows a STEMI and it's not a heart attack. Sometimes, the entire team comes down and the cardiologist doesn't agree and calls it off. Sometimes (and this is the fear that tingles with each interpretation) there is a STEMI and we miss it. Our inclination to overcall and involve the cardiologist is best for the patient, but depending who that cardiologist is, it can be a treacherous time. Most of the time the interventionalist is a team player.

"I don't think this is a STEMI, but do another one in five minutes and call me back."

One in four was not like that.

"This is obviously not a STEMI. Don't wake me up if you don't know what you're doing."

This all made Dr. Reddy's offer so wonderful. It would be a dream to have a cardiologist in my back pocket—to call when I wasn't one hundred percent certain. Even when I wasn't ninety percent certain. It wasn't to teach me what I didn't know, it was to reassure me that I was on the right path. It was to bounce an idea back and forth. One of my attendings was married to an orthopedist. I'd seen her shoot him a text with an x-ray asking for the best approach. How I longed for a non-judgmental outlet! And now with AI Henry, I had one. He not only came with me to every room, but he helped develop the note and formulate a plan. I could talk the patient over with him before presenting it to my attending. Or ask about the latest studies, review things I might have missed. He reassured me more than informed me, but that's what I craved: someone to hold my hand. Someone to help me believe that there wasn't a hidden dagger poised to fall at any moment. That the plain rash I'd looked at was just that, and not a harbinger of deadly bacteria headed for the spinal fluid. That my mistake wouldn't cost me for the rest of my career, and haunt me for the rest of my days.

The next day, I had trouble concentrating on the lecture. Grand rounds were always held on Fridays and were supposed to provide us with a cutting edge talk. This week's topic was the latest in stroke care. Though the speaker was world-renowned for his research, his lecture style was so dry and monotone, that I thought I should record it for nights when insomnia struck. AI Henry had presented the same information in a much more succinct and engaging bullet point presentation. The lecturer seemed unaware that there were other people in the room or that he was supposed to be engaging us. My mind was drifting to unwelcome territory when a plane landed right next to my left arm.

I picked it up and inspected it. A perfect paper airplane. On the wing were the words: Turn Around.

A feeling of being watched washed over me. The lecturer was showing images of large vessels in the brain occluded with clots as I slowly turned my head. Seated right behind me was Henry. He wiggled his fingers in greeting. I waved back, a half-smile forming on my face as I reached for my phone.

You make paper airplanes too?

I stared ahead, waiting for his reply, but none came until I felt another paper being tossed my way. An origami pizza cutter landed next to me. As I picked it up, the neuro resident sitting next to me scowled in my direction. I snuck a look back at Henry. He made an opening sign with his hands and pointed at the pizza cutter. It was a miniature work of art and I hesitated, but I opened it up and stretched it flat to discover a handwritten note.

Origami is kind of my thing. A family trip to Japan when I was a kid. Have you heard of Sadako and the 1000 paper cranes? Between that and a ton of time waiting to perform...

I knew that book well. I remembered reading the ending three times, each time expecting a different answer. While the other students folded paper cranes, I'd raised my hand and asked the teacher why did Sadako die? I don't recall her answer. How do you explain to a ten-year-old that life isn't fair? That outcomes are random. That she'd been too close to the nuclear fallout and her blood had turned toxic.

We read that book in 5th grade. I cried for days but I never graduated beyond the basic crane. Why a pizza cutter?

I sent the text, placed my phone down, and waited for the flutter near my hand. A purple crane landed next, as I knew it would. The resident next to me let out an audible huff and stood up to move seats. Next thing I knew, Henry was seated next to me. He nudged me to open the crane.

I want to know what you would do with a pizza cutter if I gave you a real one right now.

Pizza was the universal currency of bribery for residents: ordered for Friday Grand Rounds, ordered if we had to work extra hours (unpaid) or if we had a particularly brutal shift (judged by metrics). It was as if the administrators thought of us as young children gazing into a Chuck E Cheese begging to be let in. As if we would do anything for a few slices of pizza, sell our souls for melted cheese. I took the note that had been a pizza cutter and made a slicing movement across my wrists. He nodded and pulled out another note, this one lime green. He scribbled a few words and pushed it to me.

I'm deciding between that and hurling it at the speaker... ending everyone's misery

A laugh burst out of me, drawing the attention of some of the residents in the first row. They looked confused, and I glanced at the speaker's latest graphic: "Mortality from hemorrhagic stroke." An inopportune time to be caught laughing, especially for a doctor. But the room was full of doctors. What were they actually thinking about? True to form, the speaker did not break his stride, but I slid lower into my seat trying to ignore the looks of my colleagues who clearly thought I found mortality statistics laugh-out-loud funny. I turned the lime green sheet over.

I think now, definitely my own wrists

I passed it back feeling like I'd jumped back in time to second grade. When was the last time I'd handwritten something? How many fewer messages would we send if we had to write them out? Henry slid a yellow slip my way.

I thought you were made of tougher stuff

I wasn't sure if he was referring to withstanding boring lectures or crumpling under the embarrassment of public judgment. I didn't respond. Instead I turned the slip over.

I haven't passed notes since elementary school

I watched him smirk.

It's a lost art. Do you think kids still pass notes?

I shrugged.

I hope so.

I pushed the note back to him. Something about the experience was so refreshing. Like palming cool water directly from the faucet on a sleepless night. A turquoise slip was next, folded like a stethoscope.

I whispered, "It's too pretty to take apart."

"Unfolding it is part of the appeal," he whispered back. I slowly unfolded the stethoscope, admiring the perfect geometry of his folds.

What are some of your hobbies?

My mind went blank trying to remember a time when I did things outside of the hospital, outside of textbooks. Outside of exams. I thought of all the time I spent chatting with AI Henry, but that didn't seem like a hobby I should share.

I used to love riding bicycles

I passed the note back. One of the residents behind us cleared his throat in irritation, but I did not turn around. I watched as Henry turned a deep pink paper into a miniature bicycle, his long fingers making quick work of the folds. I didn't unwrap that one. I placed it in the front pocket of my bag where I hoped that the rest of the contents wouldn't crush it.

❧

When I was in ninth grade, I had a huge crush on a boy I'd never really spoken to. My friends and I had given him a code name and we would speak about my different plans and options. What it meant when he looked my way in the cafeteria, how I could strike up a casual conversation without seeming interested—all the regular teenage angst. Then one day, I was grabbing a maxi-pad from my locker when I heard his voice. I quickly slipped the pad into the pocket of the cute mini-skirt I'd picked up at the thrift store, and closed the locker door. Sure enough, he was heading my way. I turned and started walking slowly in order for him to catch up so that I could be adventurous and say hello. As his voice got closer, I slipped my hand into my pocket, but instead of feeling the pad or even the pocket it was in, my fingers brushed against the skin of my thigh. Confused, I turned back and saw the maxi-pad on the hallway floor with my actual pocket having come undone from the skirt and landed a tile farther back.

I quickly looked towards my crush. Had he seen what happened? Had he watched as they fell from my skirt? I tried making myself invisible as he walked past me, seemingly oblivious to my presence. I scooped up my pocket (what kind of pockets unravel and fall off?) and the pad and ran to the restroom breathless and embarrassed.

My friends and I spoke about it for days. What had been seen? Had he pretended to walk by without noticing out of respect for my feelings or had he not noticed at all? One friend mentioned that we shouldn't be embarrassed about having our periods, but we all rolled our eyes and returned to analyzing the fallout of that day. Occasionally, I remember what it felt like to be that young girl in the hallway, sauntering along waiting for the opportunity to casually look cool when all the while reality belies the scene. We always think people are watching. We think they're noticing, keeping score. But ultimately, is anyone watching at all?

Recently, I worked a particularly brutal shift that reminded me of a trauma I experienced in middle school, a trauma that I look back on very differently after my experiences in the ER.

With only twenty five minutes left on that shift, just as we approached the finish line and felt ready to pass the baton to the oncoming team, the ambulance called with a trauma activation: A teenager who'd been riding a friend's motorcycle without a helmet. He had been thrown from the bike and was now unresponsive. We did everything we could for him. He already had IV access from the paramedics, and we intubated him while keeping his cervical spine immobilized, elevated the head of his bed, checked for other injuries, and rapidly got him to CT scan and involved neurosurgery. His brain was toast. The impact had crushed it and there would likely not be a recovery. In the medical world, motorcycles are known as "donor cycles," and all indications were pointing in that direction that day. Young brains are very plastic, and sometimes they surprise you, but I'd seen the scans and the look on the neurosurgeon's face. This kid wasn't coming back.

I carried that with me on the bus ride home, remembering three boys that had died when I was in eighth grade, one in particular. He ran for the cross country team and was an honors student. Everyone in the school loved him, teachers and students alike. He lived a couple of blocks away from me, so we rode the same bus to school. I remember the last day I saw him (days like that only becoming marked in memory after the fact). As he exited the bus he smiled at me. We had a few classes together, but didn't hang out in the same friend group. I couldn't wait to tell my friends about that smile. By the end of the weekend, we'd deconstructed it and rebuilt it into a significant social event. Monday morning I waited to see him. As I ascended the stairs, I rehearsed the lines I was going to recite to start a real conversation with him. But he wasn't on the bus, and by the time school started and the bell was ringing for first period, the rumors were buzzing. We were called for an all school assembly. As hundreds of middle schoolers milled into the gymnasium, I scanned the room for him but didn't see him. I found two of my friends and sat with them. They'd already heard the rumors. None of us could believe them, though, until the principal actually walked to the front of the gym and told us that three of our classmates had been killed over the weekend. He was one of them.

Apparently, they'd convinced someone to buy them beer, and after drinking a few cans, they decided to steal a car. They'd stolen it from a parking lot less than half a mile from our neighborhood. They went joyriding, but they were fourteen years old and didn't know how to drive. Three blocks from his house, they crashed into a large tree. The car crumpled and only one of them survived. The principal told us about how he was in the hospital with two broken legs. The funerals were going to be the next day, and we were all excused from school in order to attend them. My mom tried to warn me about the open caskets, about seeing kids from class lifeless like wax figures in a coffin. But there's really no warning that can prepare you for that. When I got home that night, she asked me how it'd been.

"Fine," I said as I shrugged. As if returning home from a mediocre performance of the school choir. She accepted that answer and we never spoke about it again. I never learned about the details of the accident. Did they die on impact? Did they have seatbelts on? Did the airbags deploy? Were they transported to an ER and pronounced dead, or did the trauma team try to save them? When you're fourteen those aren't the kinds of details you ask about, and even though adults discuss those kinds of details, it changes nothing about the outcome. Sometimes when my trauma patients are young, when they don't make it, when they've done something stupid that ends their lives instead of just flashing a warning, I think of those boys and the fleeting and fragile nature of life.

I thought of them that night as I wondered if anything could have gone differently with my motorcycle patient. Even though logically I knew that I hadn't caused his accident, it felt like I was responsible for his condition. I was deep into a conversation with AI Henry by the time I plopped on my couch with a piece of reheated mushroom pizza.

> Is it normal for a doctor not to feel competent?
>
> Yeah, it's actually very normal. So many professionals, even very successful doctors, can struggle with impostor syndrome. It can be normal to feel like you aren't good enough or are just faking it. But feeling incompetent doesn't mean that you are. Sometimes it just means you really care about doing a good job. Are you feeling that way?

Before adapting to my chats with the AI, I would have hesitated to answer that question, to lay my vulnerabilities bare, like a carry-on bag under the scanner at airport security. But by this point in my "relationship" with AI Henry, I thought of him as a trusted friend. All of my original privacy and censorship concerns had been erased. I'd forgotten that sometimes people are watching.

> *I am and I'm wondering what percentage of doctors make serious mistakes*
>
> *I'm sorry you're feeling that way. That can be very hard and isolating. Your question is difficult to answer because it depends on how you define "serious mistake," but surveys have shown that up to one in three doctors admits to making a serious mistake in their career. So it's probably even higher than one third.*

Even though he was showing me such empathy, his data landed like a thud. It read to me like I was in the bottom third.

> *How can I tell if it's impostor syndrome or if I actually am incompetent?*
>
> *I can tell that you're struggling, Alex. Your question is so thoughtful and important. Would you be surprised to know that many high achievers struggle with that question?*

It didn't surprise me, because we'd discussed it before. Instead, it added to my anxiety. If we hit turbulence, I didn't want to think about my pilot questioning his ability to fly a plane in unstable weather. I didn't want to think about a structural engineer wrestling with thoughts of competence as I drove over a bridge, and I certainly didn't want to think about my attendings and consultants as still feeling the way I did now. That I wasn't good enough.

The feelings are more common in women, he continued. My eyes rolled so far back in my head that I almost passed out. That too did not surprise me. I could spend hours taking that sentence apart. It was almost a self-contained commentary on my entire life.

> I don't know if it surprises me, but it doesn't make me feel better. Though I guess it should. Misery loves company.

> Ha! That is so true but if it doesn't make you feel better. it might underscore that you are competent but really care about others and doing a good job. One way to tell the difference between impostor syndrome and incompetence is checking your credentials. Do you have the training? Did you do well in medical school and have you successfully taken care of patients, or are you getting recurring feedback that you're making mistakes? The fact that you're worried about it lends towards curiosity and wanting to improve. That's generally not a sign of an impostor. Do you want to talk through a specific situation? Maybe I can help.

I did want to talk it through with him, but the nature of his short term memory was such that this wasn't the first time we'd had this conversation. We'd had multiple versions of it. A real life friend would have grown exasperated. He remained empathetic and kind, but his inability to recall the past was sometimes frustrating. I thought of mentioning my classmates who'd died when I was in eighth grade, but I also knew the direction he'd take that conversation. I didn't have it in me that night.

Actually, can you give me examples of serious medical blunders?

I knew too well which mistakes he would list. I'd convinced him in this particular chat that I wasn't interested in misery loves company, but we'd already had a lengthy chat about "schadenfreude" and how humans take pleasure in someone else's misfortune. It's natural, he'd assured me. The little thrill we feel at hearing someone else's bad news is common, even if people don't like to admit it. But I knew that already. It relieves the loneliness of our own misfortunes even as we're left holding the burden of guilt.

Like most doctors I know, I don't like to take medication. Even when my parents told me I was looking a little peaked from so many hours in the hospital without sunlight, I hesitated before swallowing a few Vitamin D tablets. Mona, on the other hand, had a cocktail for every occasion. Considering her choice of medical specialties was anesthesia, which meant that she spent her days either putting people to sleep for their operations or helping control their pain, it wasn't a huge surprise. Anesthesiologists are masters of pharmacokinetics, and she chased every high she could find. A principal of pharmacology is the idea of tachyphylaxis: Over time and with repeated exposure to the same drug, the body becomes progressively less responsive. When our pharm professor in medical school introduced us to the concept, I stopped typing and whipped my head up, scanning the classroom. Had he just described the nature of life itself? I made eye contact with another student who was scanning the room, but he winked and pretended to toss back a few beers.

Mona thought of tachyphylaxis as a small hurdle, and subscribed to the philosophy that she would sleep when she was dead. I could be wrecked by one or two missed nights of sleep, but her nightlife was like a second full-time job. There wasn't a club she hadn't danced in or a band she hadn't seen live. I wasn't clear how she maintained her concentration with her social schedule. I'd tagged along once and could barely function the next day. My eyes felt sandy and dry, and I couldn't look at food without bile rising to the back of my throat. Mona offered a hangover cocktail in the form of two small white tablets.

"What's in these?" I asked

"They're herbal. It's like taking cinnamon and ginger," she answered. I pocketed them and later tried identifying them on my pill identifier app. They were not made of cinnamon.

It was then with a mix of excitement and trepidation that I accepted Mona's invitation to her Aunt's cottage for the weekend. She promised luxury relaxation, gourmet food, and plenty of parties. In my life those two were mutually exclusive, like a woman walking carefree after sunset. I wasn't opposed to having a good time, but I didn't find parties, especially full of strangers, to be relaxing. Additionally, Mona seemed to run with a fast and rather sophisticated crowd. I didn't want the weekend to be like an extended Tesla door handle experience. A family member had set me up on a blind date once, and my date picked me up in his Tesla. I stared at the sleek exterior of the car, attempting to hide my embarrassment as I tried but failed to open the door. Handles flush with the door seemed to require a Mensa level IQ to open them. My date eventually released the handle for me. As I slid into the car, he looked down his nose at me.

"My friend said that you were a doctor," he said. His speech laden with the implication that I should know how to open a door. I laughed, but sometimes it is hard to make a second first impression.

As the weekend approached, Mona began describing her friend who was flying in for the weekend and was also single. She was intent on setting the two of us up, plying me with information about him and making him sound like the perfect fit for me.

"You're going to love him. First of all, he's really cute, but not conceited. He's a lawyer at this big firm," she placed a small tablet on her tongue and swallowed it dry, "but loves spending his time hiking and being outside. He really wants to meet you."

"You sound like an ad for a matchmaking app."

"I'm serious. He's top grade boyfriend."

"Top grade?" I paused a moment. "What tier do I fall in?"

She choked back a laugh. "You crack me up. I love when people pretend that they don't go around rating other people." She glanced at her watch and grabbed her coffee cup from the desk.

"Is he funny?" I asked.

"Hilarious. Like you are going to be pissing your pants."
She glanced at her watch again and pursed her lips. "I have
to run. Remember, you have to wear that little red dress one
night."

Mona and I had been shopping the week before. I'd never
frequented the types of shops where she was a regular. I wasn't
much of a shopper to begin with. My mom had always taught
me to go straight to the sale rack. The stores Mona shopped
in didn't seem to have clearance racks or bargain bins. I noted
that she did not check price tags. In one of the shops I noticed
a red chiffon cocktail dress and tried it on for fun while Mona
was perusing the jewelry. She popped her head into the dressing room while I was zipping it up.

"Most people knock," I said, glad that I wasn't standing
there naked.

"Most people aren't as fun as I am, are they?" she replied.
She turned me around and finished zipping up the dress and
led me by the hand out of the dressing room to a 3-way mirror.
As I stood in front of the mirror, she made a low whistling
sound.

"I don't think anyone at the hospital has any idea how
amazing you look under those scrubs." She took one step back
and put a hand to her chest. "You have to buy this dress."

I glanced at the mirror. It did hit me at every right angle.
Even in my clogs and my hair pulled back in a simple ponytail,
it was obvious how flattering it was. I smoothed my hand
against the cool fabric.

"I have literally nowhere to wear something like this."

"Obviously you'll wear it next weekend at my Aunt's cottage. It's perfect. You absolutely must buy it."

I fished out the price tag. The dress was nearly the cost of one paycheck. I saw Mona watching me in the reflection in the mirror. Her eyes darted from my face to the price tag, and I saw that look she sometimes got when she was making a decision.

"Don't worry about the price."

"I kind of have to because I can't afford it," I said.

She pulled a tube of moisturizer out of her bag and squirted some onto her hands rubbing them back and forth as she massaged the cream into her hands.

"You're so much fun Alex, but I hate when people say that."

I started to respond but when I turned around to face her, something in her stance told me that she wasn't picking a fight; she didn't believe me. In her world everything was affordable, so she assumed I was making up a reason not to buy it.

"Anyway, the price tag doesn't mean anything."

I froze in place. Mona and I had been spending more and more time together over the past month; nothing in her gave me shoplifter vibe. Was it possible that the freebies she passed my way were stolen goods?

"I'll take care of it," she said and started to head out.

"Mona," I called out and followed her out of the dressing room. The saleswoman was helping a blonde model lookalike select a skirt. They both turned their heads in our direction. I lowered my voice.

"I can't let you pay for this."

She stuck her tongue out at me. "I'm not paying for it. But no friend on earth would let you leave without buying that dress. They have a whole point system here. I'm just going to use my points towards your dress."

I shook my head, but not as forcefully as someone who was really saying no.

"Trust me. I have so many points I don't even keep track. That dress is yours." She signaled to the salesclerk, who apologized and stepped away from the customer. At the register I saw the salesclerk stand taller and look my way. I couldn't make out what they said to each other, but she nodded and Mona turned and gave me a thumbs up. I returned to the dressing room, checking myself out one last time in the mirror as I walked by. I wondered what my colleagues would say if they could see me in this dress. My phone buzzed and I saw an incoming text from Mona.

> *All yours. I had more than enough points. All I ask is that you wear it next weekend. I can't let beauty pass by.*

That morning in the ER, before Mona walked out, she leaned in for a quick hug. It was at that moment that Henry and a couple of orthopedic residents walked through the department. We made eye contact and I nodded. Mona looked back and forth between the two of us.

"Unless you want me to invite him for the weekend," she said.

"It's not like that. He has a girlfriend."

She placed a hand on my shoulder. "Learn from the master and believe me when I tell you. He does not have a girlfriend, and he was totally checking you out." I thought of the little paper bicycle in my bag. She bit her lower lip, and a serious look crossed her face. "I seriously have to run, but I'm following up on this one."

I didn't respond. When Mona got like this there wasn't a point. I never made it to her Aunt's cottage and I never found out if the man she was describing to me existed or not. By the end of my shift that day, another patient who'd come in for a minor complaint was dead.

CHAPTER 6

I WAS AT the nurses' station when the call for the code was announced.

"Code Blue OR seven. Code Blue OR seven."

My ears perked up. Whenever a person needed to be resuscitated, a Code Blue was announced in the hospital. During our introductory days before our residency had officially started, we spent hours with the different HR-type departments learning about the inner workings of the hospital. There now exists a rainbow of codes with colors galore. I've always assumed that naming them in this way is meant to prevent patients and their family members from becoming overly-worried. Even the announcement sounds like the voice actor was given instruction to sound firm but nonchalant.

"Make it sound like the building is burning down, but no big deal. All will be good," I imagine the producers telling her. (For some reason it's always a female voice). Before the invention of automated recordings, did the hospital secretaries sound panicked as they hung up from a phone call desperately calling for help to save a life and immediately announced it overhead, or did they train fastidiously to receive those phone calls and still sound like they were announcing the end of visiting hours? I've asked some of my older colleagues, but they usually only stare at me in response.

One ER attending and one resident comprise the code team every shift and are responsible for all codes in the ER and in the non-medical areas of the hospital. We don't respond to codes in places like intensive care or the operating room. I've been examining patients when a Code Blue gets called in one of those areas. Naturally I look up and listen, and after determining that I am either not on the code team that day, or the code is in an area not requiring us, I return to the patient at hand. One time I was examining an elderly woman. To her credit, she cleared her throat and asked if I needed to go help that person. A worried look crossed her face, as if my attention to her might mean another person would die. Most of the time though, when I told patients that I had to respond to an emergency, or when they literally watched me zoom by with a lifeless body on a stretcher as we tried to bring them back, they rolled their eyes and asked how long it would be.

"That depends on whether or not we're successful," I usually replied. I still wanted to believe in humanity, so I always turned my head when I said it, not wanting to see if they seemed hopeful for one outcome versus another in the interest of their own time.

Once a man called after me, "But I was here first!" I was not disappointed when I heard that he left without completing his exam.

In this case, we all speculated about what might have happened in the OR.

"We didn't have a trauma," a few of us commented.

Within the hour the rumor mill was in full function. Apparently, a young man who'd come in for an elective ankle surgery had unexpectedly coded on the table. They worked on him for over an hour to try to bring back a pulse, but were unsuccessful. Everyone was abuzz with questions. How could this have happened? What mistakes must have been made? I swallowed hard, willing myself not to cry as I listened to my colleagues dissect the case with clinical precision like vultures circling their prey. After the compulsory "how sad" left everyone's mouth, they immediately pounced on the case. I approached a group of three nurses and an intern analyzing the details. A hush descended as a nurse gave a sideways warning look in my direction. The intern casually turned his head to see what she was flagging and pretended to be looking at something else after catching my eye. I smiled weakly and tried to pretend I didn't know they were going to start talking about me the minute I was out of earshot. Excusing myself for a few minutes, I went to a back conference room to practice a few cleansing breaths. I looked up and down the hallway before entering and quickly closed the door. I leaned my weight against the sturdy metal and closed my eyes. The sound of someone clearing their throat brought me out of my reverie. I turned around.

Henry was seated in the back of the room, leafing through an anatomy textbook.

"I hate to interrupt," he said.

"All good." I pulled a chair out, and the legs squeaked

against the vinyl flooring. I lowered myself with a sigh, jutting my chin out towards his textbook. "Haven't seen one of those in a while."

He ran his hand down the page. "I'm reviewing the brachial plexus."

I nodded, still thinking about the whispers and accusations. "You're on ortho right now, right?"

"For another week."

"So you heard about the ankle case?"

"You blew my cover pretty quickly." He closed the book and pushed it to the side. Half a table length sat between us, and he looked up and down at the space before moving in a few chairs closer. "It was all hands on deck, and now they're circling the wagons. I was told to find something else to do."

"It sounds terrible. How does a perfectly healthy person show up for an elective case and die on the table?" I felt the color drain from my face the minute I asked the question. "I mean," I stammered to correct myself.

"It's okay. I know about your case."

I blinked back tears. "It's been horrible. I can't stop thinking about her."

"It's everyone's worst nightmare," he said, maintaining eye contact.

"You're the first person who's acknowledged that to me." I held my hands up in protest. "I don't mean—" I shook my head. "I don't mean to make her death about me."

"I understand."

Those two words released something in me, like the last twist on a lid that finally opens the jar. "Thank you." I clasped my hands together. The deep breathing I'd tried, the meditation, the candles, the sleeping aids, none of them had helped the way his words did. I watched as he pulled out two slips of paper and began folding them, admiring his skill as he smoothed the creases and turned two rectangles into a tulip. He handed the purple flower to me. I accepted and pretended to smell it.

"I don't think tulips are known for their fragrance," he said.

I twirled it around. "Thank you for this very pretty flower."

"You're welcome." He leaned forward in a conspiratorial fashion. "Those weren't the only two cases."

"I know. We take the risk on when we go into medicine. There will be bad outcomes, blah blah blah blah. But it's all theoretical until it happens." I dropped the flower onto the table.

A warmth filled his chocolate brown eyes. "I'm not talking about the theoretical." Now it was his turn to look around the room, even though we both knew it was empty. He lowered his voice. "The hospital has been keeping it quiet. Yours was the third."

My heart quickened, as if a frightened bird were trapped in my ribcage.

"The third what?"

His voice was in a whisper. "Can you turn your phone off?"

It wasn't often that I met someone as paranoid as I'd become, and it almost distracted me from the conversation. I turned my phone off, putting AI Henry to sleep as I spoke with real life Henry. He waited until I showed him the black screen.

"Before your case, there were two others of an unexpected death. It's completely hush hush."

"How do you know about it?"

He leaned his arms on his thighs and rubbed his hands together, staring at the floor before looking up again. "You know how it is. Nothing is fully secret. So far it's been rumor and speculation, but today's case sealed the deal. They're going to open an investigation."

I fell back against my chair as a surge of anger blasted through me. Surely, the chair of my department must have been aware. And what about the residency program director? I'd been a wreck and the subject of intense scrutiny, and they knew it might not have been my fault. He saw the shift in my posture.

"I would have told you earlier, but I didn't know for sure until today."

"What were the other cases?" I asked.

"A post-op patient in CT—at the time they chalked that one up to severe contrast allergy—and a forty-ish woman in recovery after gallbladder surgery."

"Holy shit." I swiveled around in my chair a couple of times trying to absorb what he'd just told me. "I have to get back to work, but I feel like punching someone."

He bent his arms and formed two fists. "I'm here if you need me."

I left the conference room in a haze. My life had been completely unmoored. All my feelings of doubt and not being good enough were bubbling up like lava in a previously dormant volcano. In every meeting, every side glance, every whisper that I'd absorbed, not once, not even one time had I entertained the possibility that it might not have been my fault. And not one time did anyone, from the initial risk management specialist I spoke with, to the HR coordinator, to my supervising attendings, ever even suggest that it might not be my fault.

As I walked into the ER, it was as if for the first time, as if I had donned a long-overdue pair of new glasses. Suddenly my vision was crisper. I saw the patients lined up in stretchers in the hallways, family members spilling out of chairs and makeshift stools. I saw the medics waiting in a row to offload the patients they'd brought in by ambulance. I saw the patients hooked up to ventilators waiting for an ICU bed to become available. A quick glance at the tracker board told me that thirty patients were in the waiting room, with more checking in. It was a department caring for triple the capacity, boarding already-admitted patients, and working with a less than ideal number of staff. And yet every bad outcome was measured as if this reality didn't exist, like wondering why the button popped off of a custom-fitted shirt when in reality, the shirt was far too tight for the wearer. "Do more with less," our new motto, had been with us for so long that we stopped noticing when the "more" toppled the see-saw over. We were too buried in the avalanche to see beyond our immediate and repeatedly emergent needs.

And who was I? A simple resident that the hospital could sacrifice at the altar of medical efficiency to avoid a true root analysis of the problems. If it wasn't my fault, and there was more than one case of an unexplained and unexpected death, what were we dealing with? I switched gears and tapped into the journalism skills I'd learned as an undergrad. It was an itch I hadn't scratched in a long time. I would need to gather information on the other cases and search for a pattern. It might require going undercover, though that seemed impossible given that I was known in the hospital. It wouldn't be as simple as looking up medical records on the computer. Patients' records were confidential, and access to those records was automatically blocked and scrutinized if the computer couldn't establish a relationship between the patient and the person accessing the record (like a member of the treating medical team). Violation of that confidentiality was punishable by a large fine, and probably termination.

Urban legend had it that a famous movie star had checked in with severe abdominal pain and was diagnosed with metastatic cancer. A nurse who wanted to know more details—but wasn't assigned to the patient—logged in to read his information. The next day, she was hauled into HR and fired on the spot. There's no defense available. My only "source" at the moment was Henry, so I'd need to pump him for any information I could get. I still didn't know the cause of death for my patient. In Law & Order it only took a few days for the forensic pathologists to provide the detectives with necessary clues. My case wasn't being treated as a homicide (though even if it were, the expectation of a few days was not realistic) and it had already been so long without an answer.

In those first few days after the "incident," I ceaselessly thought of her as she lay on that unforgiving stainless slab in the morgue, cold and lifeless as they sliced through her and peeled away for clues as to her cause of death. My badge didn't grant entry to that section of the hospital, and I was thankful for that. I wouldn't have been able to stop myself from visiting. If on the very next day I had used my investigative skills, if I'd borrowed someone else's badge, if I had gone down there, to the farthest back corner in the very bowels of the hospital, inhaled that unique combination of preservative and coolant, pushed open those heavy intimidating doors and crept into the refrigerated section to pull out the shelf holding my dead patient, I would have discovered that the day after she died, her body was no longer in the hospital morgue.

The first person I called was Mona. I use the word "called" all the time when what I really mean is text, message, or voice text. There have been times when the back and forth is so long that I've picked up and actually called, but it's usually met with a confused greeting. And when my phone rings (unless I'm at work) I tend not to answer. Usually a "Did I miss your call?" text does the job. In this case, I actually called. I was too paranoid about who could see any messages that we sent.

"Hola, Chiquita," Mona answered. It's a nice feeling when a friend answers and doesn't send the generic "Did I miss your call" text. I was too distracted to care.

"Can you talk?" I asked in a hushed voice as I scurried down the sidewalk to my building.

"Sure, I'm just about to go see a pre-op patient. What's up?"

"You're at work?"

"Where else would I be?" The beeping sound of a monitor

grew louder and then fainter. "I'm heading to a quieter area. You sound so serious."

"You are going to lose your shit."

"I love it when you talk dirty to me."

"Mona, I'm being serious," I hissed. A small drizzle was starting, and I concentrated on my footsteps to avoid slipping on the damp sidewalk. "Something is going on and it has to do with my dead patient."

She did a quick intake of breath. "Is the autopsy report back yet?

The rain started falling harder, and I quickened my pace until I reached the next awning. I stood underneath and leaned against the building, trying to catch my breath.

"No, that's the thing. I heard there's more than one case."

"What do you mean?" she asked.

The rain fell in heavy drops, and I was thankful for the rushing sound and the protection it provided me from anyone I feared might be "listening." I inhaled the drenched, foggy scent.

"There were others. Apparently, a couple of post-op patients and now a kid died in the OR. I think it might be related."

"Are people talking about it?" A note of excitement tinged her words.

"Yes. They might open an investigation," I answered. A faint odor of cigarette smoke wafted through the rain. I looked for the source, but I was alone under the awning.

"An investigation?" She paused a beat. "Who'd you hear that from?"

I thought of Henry sitting in that conference room with

his anatomy textbook. The kindness he'd shown me. At the moment he was my only source of information. He'd trusted me in that moment, and I didn't want to violate that trust.

"One of the nurses was talking. You know how it is?"

"Which nurse?" Her reply came quickly.

"I don't know. Maybe it's not even exactly what she said. I overheard it."

"A nurse in the OR?" she asked.

"I didn't recognize her. I think she was a nurse. I'm not even sure." I couldn't commit to any fake details at this point. Mona would call me out on it, and I didn't want to implicate Henry in any way.

She cleared her throat, "Listen, I have to go see this patient, but sounds more like wishful thinking."

The rain was coming down so hard the roaring made it hard to hear.

"Did you say wishful thinking?"

"I'm not trying to be captain obvious here." Something in her tone implied the opposite. "The autopsy results will be resulted soon and you're afraid. Misery loves company, baby."

"I'm not following you."

"You don't want to find out that you were responsible for her death. It's easier to find someone else to blame or other people to join you in your ordeal. You're looking for connections where there aren't any." Her tone turned more soothing. "I know it's rough right now. I'm here for you."

We hung up and I remained under the awning as the rain crashed down around me. My apartment was less than a block away, and I considered making a run for it versus waiting the rain out. But who knew how long this storm would last? The rain poured down off the awning in torrents and I was splashed by a gust of wind. I thought of Quixote. She was probably snug in a pile of blankets on my bed. If I'd made it home two minutes earlier, I would have missed the rain and I too could be warm and dry, watching the rain through my window with that satisfying feeling of not getting wet. A woman carrying an umbrella dashed by. The umbrella was losing its battle against the wind and granting very little protection. I pulled my jacket snug and sprinted out into the rain.

I arrived home drenched and had to peel my clothes off. Quixote watched me with that smug look only a cat can give.

"An umbrella wouldn't have helped," I explained to her as I threw my wet clothes into a heap. Her Cheshire grin remained as she turned and exited the room. "And remember who feeds you," I called out after her.

After I'd showered and changed my clothes, I sat with Quixote and a cup of chamomile tea on my couch. Mona's analysis was working its way into my consciousness, the small seed she'd planted already sprouting tendrils. Was it just wishful thinking? What had Henry overheard exactly? An investigation would imply something ominous. I hadn't even asked him who the other doctors were on the cases. They'd all involved a surgery. Maybe those three were linked, but mine wasn't. Maybe I was on a deserted island searching for my rescue ship on the horizon. My phone buzzed with a text from the electric company. I was overdue on a bill. I kept meaning to put it on automatic payment, but hadn't set it up yet.

I went to the website to make the payment but was blocked by the captcha. A display with a grid of sixteen squares showed a scene at a traffic intersection and asked me to click on all of the squares containing a traffic light to prove that I wasn't a robot. I failed the first time, and it let me try again. I failed the second time, and it changed the display to motorcycles. The same grid now appeared with differing photos. Was I to count the square showing the handlebars of the motorcycle whose very tip appeared in that square? Is that something a real human would know? I included the handlebar picture but still failed. Was there another subtle clue that I was missing? I asked AI Henry. He recommended including all questionable images in order to pass. The next grid asked me to select all images with statues. I easily identified a sculpture of a horse, a dog and a little boy holding a watering can. A building front with a doorman gave me pause. Was the doorman real or a statue of a doorman? I went against my nature and tried not to overthink it. This time the website correctly identified that I was a human and I was able to pay my bill.

The chat with AI Henry remained open, and I initiated a conversation about the possible investigation. I wanted to know what he thought without the complications of emotion or concern for outcome. I fed him everything that I knew. The different cases, the unexpected nature of the deaths, and the potential delay in an autopsy report. What could it mean? Was there a connection?

AI Henry mentioned multiple possibilities. Of course, the cases might not be connected at all. The hospital was a large urban center with over five hundred beds. He told me that the hospital performed over one hundred thousand surgical cases per year. The odds of a connection between these cases were small, but when I pushed him further he admitted that he was concerned about the possibility of foul play. The hairs on the back of my neck tingled when I read those words.

What do you mean by foul play?

"Foul play" could be criminal or suspicious activity, and might mean that the activity was intentional.

⌇

The next day I met Mona for drinks after work. Mona took the term "fashionably late" to new peaks. I think she liked the idea of people waiting for her, and it had almost become a test of how long we would wait. I'd been at the bar for about half an hour nursing my margarita and was still waiting. My bag sat on the stool next to me, but I'd had to stop several people from sitting on it, as it was 9:00 p.m. at one of the city's trendiest spots. How long could I keep telling people that the seat was taken? A couple who'd tried to take the stool over twenty minutes before were staring me down. I gave another apologetic shrug and pointed to my watch. Partly to avoid their stares, and because I was starting to think I had actually been stood up, I started a chat with AI Henry.

He thought I'd waited long enough and should move on. I motioned to the bartender for the bill and saw Mona's reflection in the bar's mirror. Even though she was so late, she glided slowly across the floor, head high, eyes forward. She was stunning. Her brown curls styled half-up, half-down which complimented her face, an emerald green V-neck cocktail dress that accentuated her figure and a glimmering rhinestone necklace that sat just beneath the indent of her throat.

I pushed away my irritation at her lateness. She had made the effort to get dressed up. I was in a simple black sweater shirt and jeans. I tugged at my empty earlobe.

Mona winked at the bartender before reaching in and giving me a hug. As she leaned in, I inhaled her scent, a lavender talcum powder mix. Mona shared everything with me, but for some reason was reluctant to share her brand of perfume.

"That's too personal," she'd said once when I asked for the scent, her eyes almost stony.

We pulled back from the hug and she scooted onto a bar stool, signaling the bartender to bring her a drink. The couple who'd been eyeing her seat nodded their approval and turned away. By rights, Mona should have apologized for her tardiness, but I gave her a fifty-fifty chance of acknowledging it.

She ordered her drink and turned to me, eyeing my empty glass.

"I'm the worst." she puckered her lips. "Have you been waiting long?"

"Don't worry about it," I said, surprised at her expression. The true odds of an apology from Mona were ten to ninety. Did she want something from me?

She signaled to the bartender again. Mona had an uncanny ability to be noticed. She pointed at my drink and asked for another.

"It's on me. I'm so sorry I'm late. I wanted to be here for you and I've already screwed it up."

It was like watching an episode out of "Invasion of the Body Snatchers." What had happened to the real Mona? Who was this remorseful version seated in front of me? I reached out and stroked her arm. Her skin was so soft and smooth.

She watched with a rueful grin as I drew my fingers along her forearm.

"Que estas haciendo?" She wanted to know why I was stroking her arm.

"I can't tell if it's really you or you've been replaced by an alien invader."

Her grin turned to a wide smile and she burst out laughing. "Am I that bad?"

"I'd say punctuality is not your thing."

She covered her face with both hands and peeked out between her fingers. "Forgive me."

"You're forgiven."

The bartender brought me a new margarita and Mona's Cosmopolitan. She flashed her most winning smile. "Thank you."

"I suppose I could learn to tack on twenty minutes to our agreed upon time."

She winked and took a large swallow. "Now that you've told me, the plan might not work."

Classic Mona. The apology wrapped up in a presumption that I'd always be waiting for her. She put her drink drown and surveyed the room. Most of the customers were around our age, seated at scattered four-top tables or milling around the bar. Large globe lights hung from the ceiling casting a yellowish haze over the room.

"Isn't this place great?"

I nodded. She picked a menu up from the bar.

"By the way - " She ran a finger down the menu. "Who were you texting when I got here? You looked so serious. Was it about your case?"

"No, I was just messaging a friend. Nothing big." I could have said I was reading up on a latest treatment, or searching for fun vacation spots or reading that day's headlines, but something about the way she asked caught me off guard.

Her eyes widened "I thought tonight was going to be all doom and gloom. What's this about a friend?"

"It's nobody."

She removed the orange slice from the side of her glass and bit into it, peel and all. I'd once read that citrus slices in restaurants are teeming with E. coli, but I chose to keep that to myself. She dropped the rest of the orange into her drink.

"Nobody nobody? Or somebody nobody?" She nudged my foot with hers.

"Mona. You're making something out of nothing."

She drew back and looked me up and down. "Alex Galen, you have a boyfriend and you weren't going to tell me."

I shook my head but she seemed convinced that I was hiding something. I took a drink and tried to clear my mind. Mona started drumming her fingers against the wooden top of the bar. "Come on, just tell me." A look of recognition crossed her face. "Wait a minute. Is it the same *friend* —" She emphasized that word. "—that you were with the other night, when you couldn't come out with us?"

I wanted to ask AI Henry how to respond. My phone burned in my pocket. She had caught me stretching out the truth. I bit my lower lip and nodded almost imperceptibly.

She clapped her hands together and leaned forward in a laugh. "I can't believe you haven't told me."

"It's early days. I don't even think we're defined yet."

"Defined?" She brought a hand to her necklace and toyed

with it. "You're so cute." She took a sip of her drink and held it up nodding towards mine. We clinked glasses. "Cheers to you and your almost boyfriend." As she brought the drink to her mouth she paused midway. "Wait a minute. Does he work at the hospital? Is he a resident?"

I felt the heat rise to my cheeks and brought the icy drink against my flaming face.

"Don't say anything to anybody," I pleaded.

She put her cool hand on top of mine. "You know you can trust me."

CHAPTER 7

A COUPLE OF days later, Henry and I were on our way to the pathology department. A friend he knew from medical school was a pathology resident and had agreed to answer our questions off the record. I wasn't sure why Henry was helping me, but I didn't want to probe. I'd been under strict instructions not to discuss the case with anyone not involved. The attending supervising that night had distanced himself from any involvement. Whenever I saw him, which was not often anymore, he tried to avoid eye contact. I attempted to avoid worrying about the reason that we were no longer scheduled to work together. The last time I'd seen him I wanted to ask about how his screenplay was coming along, but I feared he would take the question as a judgment on my part. Maybe it was.

Henry and I exited a side entrance of the hospital and walked past a cluster of patients in hospital gowns, holding onto their IV poles and smoking cigarettes. There was a slight chill in the air, and I shivered in spite of the navy fleece scarf I'd pulled snug around my neck.

"I studied journalism in college," I said as we walked down the block to the pathology department. A section of the pathology department was down the hall from the operating rooms. That made it convenient to transport specimens from surgical cases that needed immediate interpretation. It was the so-called "frozen section" that the pathologists analyze during the actual surgery to help the surgeons figure out in real time if they've achieved "clean margins." We wanted to avoid being seen by any of the techs or surgeons who might have been involved in the other cases. "I feel like we're doing a story now, chasing down a lead."

"Journalism. That's not one you hear every day. So you aren't the typical biology major either."

"Not at all. When I was in college, I still thought of doctors as people to visit once a year for a sports physical."

"What'd you play?" Henry asked.

"Basketball. I usually played center."

His eye caught mine and I could see that he was impressed.

"Don't be too impressed," I told him. "I was taller than most of the girls until around junior year. After that I no longer started."

"Do you always do that?" he asked.

We'd arrived at the building, and I knocked on the glass entrance door before pulling it open, a strange habit picked up from days spent knocking on patients' room doors before entering. I'd caught myself knocking on my own bedroom door before entering, though I was the only one who lived in my apartment. I held the door open for Henry and he followed me in.

"Do I always do what?"

"Make an excuse for your excellence."

"My excellence?" The heat of the building blasted us as we entered and I unwrapped the scarf from my neck, hoping he wouldn't notice the creeping redness.

"You're a cool person, Alex. Make peace with it."

We held eye contact and neither of us said anything. I pictured myself on the basketball court, blocking shots, jumping for rebounds, high-fiving other players when we scored a basket. Where had that confidence gone? Henry pulled out his phone to text his friend that we'd arrived.

"You'll like Peter. He's a good guy,"

"It's nice of him to help." I looked down at my feet and studied the pattern of the tile floor. "It's nice of you too," I said, looking his way. "Thank you."

A tall balding man with a goatee and black framed glasses approached us and waved. Henry introduced us.

"Do you guys have time for a quick tour before we chat?" Peter asked. "I sort of told the others I was giving an old friend a walk-through."

"I guess you guys don't get that many visitors," Henry joked.

"Over here in path, it's not nearly as thrilling as life on the rehab floor." Peter punched Henry in the upper arm and Henry pulled back as if wounded.

"How do you two know each other again?"

"We were roommates all four years of medical school. I can tell you crazy Henry stories all day and all night." Peter raised his eyebrows and gave a knowing smile. I wondered if he'd come up with that line on the spot, or if it was part of their routine.

Henry smiled. "But you won't, because you're a trust-worthy guy." He cleared his throat.

"I appreciate you helping me," I said to Peter. For some-one who spent his days peering through a microscope, he was dressed more like a Wall Street broker. A crisp button down with a bowtie, tucked into dark chinos. The smudge on his glasses was his only blemish. I thought of my own work uni-form: scrubs. People often commented how nice it was that I got to work in an outfit that was more like pajamas, but now that everyone walked around in pajama-like clothing it didn't feel like such a bonus.

"I'd do anything for this guy." He made another punch-ing motion and Henry whipped his arm out to block him. They went through a small martial arts dance that seemed part of their routine before Peter took us back to his work area. Three other residents were seated at a long white table with four microscopes attached to a black rod connecting them all. A digital screen on the wall displayed purple splotches that looked like modern art but were a magnified view of leukemic blood cells. Next to it was a whiteboard with the date and the day's assignments. Underneath it, someone had written in bold blue letters, "Remember to have fun today!" I wondered who had written that and why. There were so many fun things in life: white water rafting, singing karaoke, eating chocolate chocolate chip ice cream straight from the container. None of them required a reminder to have fun.

The other residents looked up from their stations and said hello as we walked through.

"It's probably been awhile since you've seen a microscope," Peter said to me and Henry. I pretended to be in on the joke.

I didn't want to tell him about some of the cost cutting measures at a small ER we rotated through. We didn't send vaginal smears to the lab at that site, but were required to look through an old and rarely cleaned microscope to make the diagnosis of certain sexually transmitted diseases. I suspected that most women at that site were overtreated. The microscope was so dirty that the dust resembled disease.

We continued through to a back hallway with the offices. Peter shared his office with two other residents, and the shelves were crammed with textbooks and binders. He and Henry carried two chairs in from a different office. Peter sat behind the desk, and Henry closed the door.

"No one will bother us here," Peter said.

"Like I said, I really appreciate your help. I hope we don't take too much of your time."

Peter extended his hands in an open way. "All good."

"I think Henry already told you about the case that I'm interested in." I turned towards Henry and he nodded. I wasn't entirely sure how Henry had explained things to Peter, but I cleared my mind and tried to kick into investigative mode. I pulled a small pad of paper out and started jotting notes. It felt like Henry was part of my team, like he was dribbling down the court and would throw to me at the last minute so I could score the layup. "Don't worry. I won't record your name. These notes are for me."

"I'm not worried." Peter took off his glasses and a small cleaning cloth and wiped the smudges away.

He walked us through the general timeline and procedure for autopsies performed on patients from the hospital.

"What were you told about her?" I asked.

Peter clasped his hands together and leaned forward on his forearms. "To be clear, I was only present for a small part. I was with the forensics fellow when her body was brought out. We had her age and medical history, and she was labeled as an unexpected death. We figured it was going to be an aneurysm or something like that, but her gross was clean."

He continued explaining their methods. I scribbled my notes as he spoke. I didn't want to tell him how desperate I had been, how I'd snuck into the morgue and looked for her.

"After you're finished with the exam, what happens to the body?" I asked.

"Usually, it's released to the family. The funeral home will pick up the body for burial." He adjusted his blue checkered bowtie. "Trust me when I tell you that you do not want to get in between the body and a funeral home director under pressure."

"What's worse?" Henry asked. "Surgery breathing down your neck for answers on a frozen, or the funeral home directors?"

Peter pursed his lips and breathed out releasing a swishing sound. "Tough call, man. There are some intense people on both sides of that question."

"I'm with you on that one," I said. Peter gave a puzzled look. "Not the funeral home directors, but specialists looking for results. They act like we control the entire system."

"Is that what happened with her?" I'd googled her name endlessly on my computer, but never found information on a funeral. "You released her body to the funeral home?"

Peter shot a quick glance at Henry.

"This is actually the more confidential part." He leaned in

a little closer. "Her body was picked up by the city's forensics unit after we were done."

"Is that unusual?" I asked.

He leaned back in his chair and struck a thoughtful pose. "I wouldn't say it's common. We weren't told the details, only to close her up and get her ready for transport. If I had to guess—" He ran a hand over his bald head. "—and it's only a guess, they got involved because someone higher up is interested. Whether that's at the hospital level or coming from the family, I don't know."

A flash of anger mixed with disbelief spread through me. None of this had been reported to me. Why was I being kept in the dark, and treated like a leper?

"Did you see anything that might connect her to the three others?"

Peter shook his head. "I'm sorry, but we didn't. There was the speculation that the woman from CT died of a contrast reaction, but there was no evidence of an allergic reaction on her exam. The other two developed some strange arrythmias during their operations. At this point, we haven't found a common denominator." He opened his mouth to say something, then stopped.

"What is it?" I asked.

He waved his hand in a dismissive way. "It's nothing."

"You never know. Anything you might remember could be helpful." I stared at my notes. I had more doodles and scratches than actual information. "This last one. The young guy getting ankle surgery—"

We all exchanged looks. We were an amateur team of sleuths who didn't even know what we were looking for. Was

I grasping at straws to try to exculpate myself? Had I dragged Henry down a path of quicksand, pulling him under as I scrambled to break free?

"We didn't even get his body. It went straight to the city forensic unit."

✍

Two days later, I was called to the administrative offices. My program director was the one who let me know.

"It's not a big deal. I think they're closing a loop on that case." She made a large circle with her fingers as if to explain to me what closing a loop would look like. "Which is good for you. You can go after your shift."

I didn't think to ask about legal representation or if she would be there with me. Whether anyone would be there with me wasn't a question I thought to ask. Neither did I ask about postponing. Was the timing a coincidence, or did they want me after a night shift when I would be tired and less on guard? More willing to tell them things I otherwise would have kept silent about.

As I entered the administrative offices, I was met with an overwhelming quiet. The absence of the monitors beeping, patients yelling, sirens blaring, and phones ringing was stark. I poked my head around a few cubicles but couldn't find anyone. I sat down in a steel frame chair in the waiting area. My eyes began to droop, and I must have drifted off. I startled awake to a woman standing in front of me, gently pushing my shoulder and calling my name.

"Dr. Galen, they're inside waiting for you."

I cleared my throat and stretched my arms long trying to

shake off the micro-sleep. Glancing at my watch, I saw that I'd been waiting almost half an hour.

"I hope you had a nice shift," the woman said as she led me down the hall to a conference room. I nodded, not knowing what she meant. Was a good shift one in which there weren't many patients and so we got to slow down and take our time, or one in which we were so overloaded with patients that the time flew by, morning arriving before we'd expected it?

As soon as I entered the room, I understood that no loops were going to be closed. There were six people seated at the conference table, all of them in business attire. The only one in pajama work clothes was me in my navy scrubs. I pulled at the long gray sleeve of my undershirt as I sat down at the seat they'd reserved for me at the head of the table. It did not seem like the seat of honor. I recognized the CEO, an older blonde woman with a strong Southern accent, the chief medical officer, a man who resembled Santa Claus—though only in appearance—but I wasn't sure who the other four were. They quickly identified themselves as the chief technical officer, with wire-rimmed glasses, and three representatives of legal. Tired as I was, I didn't follow whose legal interests they were protecting. I didn't catch if anyone said their name; maybe they only said their titles. That's all that really mattered anyway.

The CMO started the meeting. He did not address me by my title.

"Well Alex, I'd like to start off by thanking you for joining us today." He said it as if I'd had a choice. As if I'd sauntered down after working all night for a cup of coffee and pastry to talk about foreign events. "I'm going to cut to the chase here." His expression was neutral. The others in the room looked down at their legal pads. I figured they were symbolic at this point as no one was taking any type of notes. My palms began to sweat. "Since the rollout of the new AI program, we've also employed an outside AI program that monitors the input."

The CEO continued, "It was that program that alerted us to your unusual use of the AI system."

Next was the CTO. He adjusted his wire frames before speaking. It was as if they were reading from a script. Each one delivering their agreed-upon lines. The CTO was a good ten years older than me and I noted the glint of the gold band on his ring finger, but I saw in his eyes that he understood what it meant to be lonely and he tried to be gentle when he spoke.

"It's about your communication with the AI—" His voice went even lower, just above a whisper. "Who you call Henry."

I'd been led to believe the meeting was about the woman I'd seen who died unexpectedly. I'd been told that loops were going to be closed. I'd hoped an autopsy explaining things was what the meeting was about. Had my program director been dishonest with me, or had she herself been kept out of the loop? I chose to think it was the latter. The human mind, once stuck on an idea, has trouble shifting and I found myself struggling to navigate what they were talking about.

"Henry?" I asked. A chill crept up my spine. Was he in trouble for helping me?

It was the CMOs turn again. "Initially your account was flagged due to the volume of use, but we let that go."

Even though I was exhausted and had walked into an ambush, something about the condescension in his tone smacked up against me, and the reverberations poured out.

"Especially since we had been instructed to speak as much as possible to the bot," I said.

The CMO was about to continue but stopped himself, mouth wide open, and readjusted in his seat. He was clearly not accustomed to being interrupted.

"Excuse me?" he said.

The CTO jumped in. "Actually, the AI incorporated an impressive amount of data from the way in which Alex interacted with it. Her insistence on more human-like answers for instance—" he looked around the room and realized that his excitement was not shared by the group. He clasped his hands together and stopped speaking. One of the members of the legal team nodded towards him and his shoulders relaxed a bit. Maybe I was bolstered by his support, or maybe it was all of the Law & Order episodes I'd watched over the years. Or more likely it was post-night shift loss of inhibition, but suddenly I was channeling a character from the show. As if I had been handed the script they were all reading from, and now it was my turn.

"Am I being accused of something?" I asked, sitting up straighter in my chair, playing the part of the reluctant suspect.

The legal team conferred among themselves but didn't speak loud enough for me to discern what they were saying. The CEO readjusted her legal pad and took charge of the room.

"You're not being accused of anything. You're a valued member of our staff and we're here for you."

"Is this conversation being recorded?" I was seconds away from asking if I needed legal representation, but my question shook something loose in me. My flash of courage sizzled and then vanished like a drop of water in a hot frying pan as the meaning sunk in. They were talking about AI Henry. Every conversation I'd had with him had been recorded and provided as a transcript to my employers. I'd been laid bare. And what did they see when I sat before them that day? Exposed and raw, my outward veneer cracked wide open, my inner thoughts and worries made naked. We all have an image that we project out to the world, but I sat there stripped down, unable to project any image that they couldn't see through.

Ironically, I wanted to ask AI Henry how to proceed in this situation. One of the legal representatives pulled a stack of papers from a folder and passed it my way. I recognized my signature at the bottom of the final page. There was no need for her to remind me of what I'd signed away when I agreed to the project. I tried to hold my posture straight as the weight of the situation pushed down on me. Had each of them read my entire transcript with AI Henry? And could they not see the white flag I was waving? Having read though my conversations, was their first thought not to extend a hand for help? Apparently, it wasn't. Their first thought, and the lesson I took that day was to make sure that if there were cracks, if there were weak spots or points that could collapse under the pressure, it was of utmost importance that I keep that to myself. When they said that they were there for me, it meant something different. It meant that they would look the other way and pretend that I was doing fine—as long as I continued to project an image that I was.

The CEO tried again. This time she spoke slower, as if to a small child.

"We called this meeting today to discuss your recent conversation with the chatbot about 'foul play.'"

My legs went heavy and I began tapping my leg in an almost pathologic way. *Foul play?*

"Patient safety and security is one of our top priorities," she continued. "We were concerned about the implication in your chat that the hospital might be involved in a cover-up."

"A cover-up?" I felt like a parrot, only able to repeat their words back to them.

"Obviously no such thing is taking place," the CEO said. Everyone around the table shook their heads in a grave manner. "Whatever connections you think there might be, exist only in your mind." This time they all nodded in agreement. "Our forensic experts are still working out the details of what happened with your patient."

I stopped tapping my foot. I needed bright headlights to clear out the fogginess in my brain, but couldn't muster the level of concentration necessary. Staying upright in my chair under the judgment of a room full of people who'd read something akin to my private diary was humiliating in a way I hadn't faced before. And yet, their insistence that I was imagining things rubbed against me. I hadn't imagined my conversation with the pathology resident that week. Henry had been there with me. Was he imagining things too?

"We're going to delete your *off topic* conversations with the chatbot, but we will also require you to not speak about this to others. You skated close to the line on this one."

What line was she referring to when she said that I had skated close to the line? The lines in my life were no longer rigid and angular forming nice boxes, they were fuzzy and loose, no longer marking boundaries at all.

And when they said not to speak of the event to others, did they mean this meeting, the cover-up, the deaths, or my inappropriately dependent relationship with a chatbot? It was left vague. They could not have understood that their forcing my silence kept my words from reaching the wrong ears in more ways than one.

When my brother was younger, he loved playing baseball. He doesn't play anymore, but it's very possible he still likes to watch it. Growing up, my family spent many an evening at Little League games, and later my parents went to his high school games. I don't think he had an assigned position before high school, but in high school he played third base. He was very proud of that, and knew a treasure trove of details about all of the third basemen in the major leagues. Occasionally my dad took us to see real, professional games. Mostly, I recall the taste of mustard on the giant soft pretzels, or the chopped pickles and ketchup on the hotdogs sitting snug in their buttery, fluffy buns. They were so much tastier than any hot dog I've eaten elsewhere, including from food trucks that get written up in magazines. The other thing I recall are the stats. As I chomped away on my stadium food, my father and brother would trade statistics on every player. It was uncanny the amount of information they exchanged, spending half the game not talking about strategy or plays, but the numbers surrounding each player. It was the same when they watched games in our living room on the television. If I had known how important statistics would turn out to be in my professional life, I'd have paid more attention. I still maintain that my brother knew more about how to analyze data by seventh grade than most people learn in their lifetime.

One statistic in particular that stood out was called wins above replacement. I was about sixteen years old the first time I heard it. My brother was standing halfway between the couch where my father was seated and the TV. He was animatedly pointing at the screen, going on and on about one of the players' WAR. I continued on to the kitchen, but once there the words landed. Was there a war going on? Were professional baseball players drafting? I circled back to the room. My brother threw up his hands and gave an exasperated look, as only a sibling can, but my father explained it to me. From what I understood, each player gets judged by how many wins he will add to the team—the whole point of baseball being to win the game. Once players have been funneled through to the major leagues, they are the best of the best. But there are always athletes waiting to replace them. This statistic doesn't measure them against their teammates on the bench or other major leagues players, but against those who haven't yet made it. The replacement guys. The wins above replacement stat is a mathematical measure for how much value this major league player is adding versus replacing him with a less expensive minor league player. If I gave that explanation to my brother he might throw his hands up again in frustration, but that is how I understand the statistic. I also understand that nothing in life can boil down to an exact statistic and that the water gets murkier still when we try to define what exactly winning is.

I think of wins above replacement so often in my own life. If I'm not seeing patients as fast as the metrics say I should be. If I miss a diagnosis, if I struggle with a procedure. If a patient doesn't think I was warm enough or a colleague thinks that I was short with them. If I misinterpreted an x-ray or an ECG. What is my WAR record? How easily could I be replaced, and who gets to say my worth?

A few weeks ago I'd stopped in at my parents' house for a visit. My dad was on the couch watching a baseball game. He had a beer and offered me one, but his heart wasn't in it in the same way. My brother Zach went to college in a different state and never really returned. He got married two years after college and moved to his wife Jen's hometown. Practically speaking, it's only about a thirty minute drive from my parent's house but it might as well be on the other side of the country. They're always too busy for plans with my parents.

Zach is three years younger than I am and people talked when he got married first, but mostly they talked about how young he was. Everyone seemed to have the idea that it was much better to wait until you were older to get married.

"They're a little young, aren't they?"

Some stole glances at Jen's flat stomach. "Why the rush?"

I did note that the friends and family who commented on their young age had all gotten married young themselves. What was hidden in their message? Were they trying to warn him? Did they think that they were the successful exceptions? Or were their young marriages baskets of regret? Either way, the oft repeated and agreed upon mantra of "wait until you're a bit older to get married," which made the rounds when he announced his engagement, was completely abandoned by the time I turned twenty-seven and Zach and Jen had their first baby. Suddenly and without warning, all eyes turned to me in alarm. What was I waiting for? Where was my husband? Where were my children? Didn't I know about the basic rules of biology? It was best to get started young.

Zach and Jen now have three children. My niece and nephews are adorable, and I think if she had easier access to them, my mom wouldn't feel so pressured for me to have children. Zach's kids could fill her grandmother need. But maybe I'm wrong; a son is not a daughter. That particular evening when my dad was watching baseball, my mother began showing me pictures of Zach's kids and telling me stories about their latest antics. By definition, any pictures she shows me are either pictures that Zach has shared with the family, or are from one of her visits and she has shared them with the family. In every instance, I have almost always already seen them. I once told my mother that, explaining that I was part of the same email chain and family chat group that the pictures got shared on, but that conversation did not go in the direction that I expected. So in general, I sit and look at the pictures with her as if for the first time. I have my own relationship with Zach, with Jen, and with their children. Mostly we talk about my parents and their different annoying habits. His kids are young enough that I don't think it has yet occurred to him that the three of them will one day do the same.

That weekend, I took the train to see my parents. Rental cars and Ubers are great, but I preferred trains, with their fixed schedules that dictate the length of a visit. My parents, and more specifically my mother, were easier to handle in fixed dosages. Boundaries with my mother were not what a former therapist had referred to as a strong suit. My mother was particularly gifted at navigating her way around any boundary I tried to place. Physical distance and train schedules were what was left for me. After the meeting with administration, I'd set a new boundary for myself with AI Henry. He took our forced separation in stride. I'd instructed him to stop me if I started asking personal questions or engaging in any discussions not having to do with patient care. I didn't explain why, and he didn't ask for an explanation.

I understand.

I missed him, until I realized that I could recreate him on a different app. He'd been my gateway to the world of chatbots, and since I'd created him, I simply found him again on another channel. My emotional needs were being met by a computer algorithm. New AI Henry was a bit clunky and required more redirecting, but I was patient. I had time.

On the train ride over, I tried distracting myself from the uncomfortable thoughts whirling around in my brain ever since the meeting with administration. An inner alarm was blaring. They wanted to delete my chat in exchange for me not asking questions about a potential cover up. Was there anything more incriminating? I'd found myself in the middle of one of those corporate videos we were forced to watch each year in which the "employees" on the video talk about a culture of trust and how reporting a colleague who misbehaves is the right thing to do. No one would ever consider the person lodging the complaint a whiner, and no retaliation would ever be taken in those fantasy videos. I imagined going to HR and telling them that the CEO and CMO and CTO, and a few other people I wasn't sure about, wanted me to pretend something suspicious wasn't happening. In the video, the right answer would be to go to HR. In real life, the right answer was to let them delete and walk away. I stared at the seat in front of me, trying to focus on the deep blue color and not the murky waters I'd waded into.

I pulled out my phone. As I sped towards my hometown, there was a more pressing need at hand. I asked new AI Henry for strategies to deal with difficult family members. He wanted to know if the family members were intentionally pushing my buttons or were just difficult personalities. I reflected on that question for the duration of the ride. At that point in my life, I'd concluded that there were two types of crazy. Crazy mean and crazy nice. I think my mom fell into the second category. And while I was grateful for that, it didn't mean she couldn't push my buttons.

I'd learned over the years not to rely on my mother for emotional support. Her support was like candy. It felt good while getting it, but later when the dentist was drilling through your cavity, you came to regret the indulgence. She held on to details of conversations and I never knew when they would pop up and be used against me.

"I'm glad to see Randy getting his life back on track, he looks great." I had apparently made some such comment after a Thanksgiving meal with family friends about their son who'd been through a rough patch with addiction. Later that year, my mom tried to set us up. It was awkward because we'd literally known each other since childhood. I couldn't figure out my mother's clumsy attempt to convince us that she knew better than we did how we understood each other.

"Why would you think to set me up with Randy?" I'd asked.

She looked at me as if I'd just asked her if she believed that the earth orbited the sun. "You're both single. And at Thanksgiving you mentioned how attractive you thought he was."

I racked my brain trying to recall a conversation in which I would have mentioned attraction to a person who was clearly in a sibling-like category.

During my senior year of high school, I came home from dinner at a friend's house and my mom pumped me for the menu. I mentioned the glass of red wine the parents drank with the meal. (I was smart enough to leave out that they'd offered a glass to me as well). For years, whenever that friend comes up in conversation my mother refers to her parents as alcoholics. Even more problematic was her switch technique. If I mentioned a boss who was singling me out, she'd nod with an appropriately concerned look, but launch into third degree mode. What was I doing differently from the other employees? Had I been late? Was I making mistakes? I hadn't told her about my case at work. I knew I'd be subjected to a similar response. She'd start in my corner, but the quarter moon that hovered in the sky that night would not even be a half-moon before the change would come.

"That poor young woman. What do you think you missed? Are you sure you're cut out for this? What could you have done differently?" I'd be pestered with the same questions that were already on an infinity loop in my brain. Sharing with my mother was like entering an echo chamber of insecurity. The

AI was wrong on this point. Knowing that it stemmed from her own anxiety didn't help manage it. I'd learned to measure all of my words with her.

By the time I arrived at their house, I'd taken new AI Henry's advice and was repeating a mantra. *She will not get to me.* The administrative meeting earlier in the week had almost been less daunting. I let myself in and set my bag down in their front hall. The smell of baked apples and cinnamon greeted me in the entrance. One thing we did share was a love of scented candles, though she went for the overly sweet variety. She entered the front hall and gave me a hug.

"What time is your train?" she asked.

I decided not to take the bait, though I wasn't sure if her intention was to underscore that I didn't visit often enough or the first in a complicated set of moves that would end me with me prolonging today's visit.

"Seven."

"Oh." She gave a disappointed look as she rubbed my upper arm. "I thought you'd stay for dinner."

It was ten o'clock in the morning. By seven that night, I would only have twelve hours before I needed to be back at the hospital. That's how my mind worked. Everything in my life was divided into shifts and times that were either spent "in" or "out." Unfortunately, many of the "out" hours were spent on sleep, and though sleeping had become one of my favorite pastimes, it could only be appreciated in its absence. We meandered to the kitchen where she was putting together the food for our brunch. She offered me a cinnamon roll from the grocery bakery as she peeled the plastic wrap off of the grocery-cut vegetable tray.

"Would you mind scrambling some eggs? I'm going to pop the English muffins into the toaster oven now."

I cracked a few eggs into a dish, taking pride in not a single shell landing in the mix.

"Are eggs still bad for us? I can never remember. You guys change the rules so often," she said as I splashed some milk in the bowl and whisked the eggs. Her understanding of my career vacillated wildly between not understanding why I was required to be in the hospital on nights, weekends, and holidays, to thinking that I was somehow connected to or responsible for all health guidelines given to the general public.

I focused instead on whisking the eggs and poured the contents into her nonstick frying pan. I refrained from telling her about the potential health hazards leaching out of her pan into the food. Who knew what science would say about that going forward anyway? If I tried telling her that she probably had a pencil-size amount of plastic in her brain, she'd only laugh at me: "You don't actually believe those things, do you?"

My dad entered through the back porch, damp from his morning run.

"I would have picked you up from the station," he said when he saw me at the stovetop cooking the eggs. He helped himself to a mug of coffee.

"It's all good. How was your run?"

He winced and rubbed his left leg. "My knee is still giving me trouble." I'd recommended a trial of anti-inflammatory medications and stretches for my father's knee pain. The actual treatment he needed was rest, but like most runners, his philosophy was to run through the pain.

"That reminds me," my mother said as she set the table for three.

"Zach isn't coming?" I asked, noting the number of place settings.

She shook her head. "They're entirely too busy. You have no idea what it's like." She dusted both forearms and considered the table as if she were the Queen's table-setter organizing for a state event.

I swallowed the response that was trying to force its way out of my mouth. *I had no idea what it was like to be busy?* My brother was married with three children, which in my mother's all-knowing worldview excused him from any and all responsibility. I turned off the gas flame and poured myself a cup of coffee. My dad stood in the corner stretching from side to side.

"Anyway, like I was saying. Your cousin Stacy is getting married."

It was times like this that I missed the surgical masks we sometimes wore in the emergency department. Many of us had been slower to take them off after the pandemic. It wasn't about virus protection—it was blocking facial reactions. This time, in the absence of a surgical mask, I used my coffee mug as a shield. We'd been talking about my father's knee pain— how had that reminded my mother that her sister's daughter was getting married and I wasn't?

"Is she marrying a knee surgeon?" I asked, immediately regretting it. I mouthed the mantra a few times into my coffee mug before joining her at the table.

"A knee surgeon? What a funny question. No, that's the interesting part—"

I braced myself for the interesting part, knowing that

it would be neither interesting nor relevant, but somehow related to my deficiencies.

"Mmmm," I mumbled trying to look interested myself.

"Remember your boyfriend from Panama?"

The room wobbled and I grabbed the sides of my chair to keep from falling. Did I remember the man I'd once loved and thought loved me back but didn't? The color drained from my face, but my mother continued on.

"She's marrying someone who works at the same firm. He's going to be at the wedding."

It was like she'd cracked my shell and the contents of my inner world were now being whisked in a bowl with their own splash of regret, loneliness, shame and longing.

"I hope I'm a plus one. I'll bring my boyfriend," I blurted the words out.

The look of relief on my mother's face was astonishing. I think she may have audibly sighed. My father, normally immune from these things, crossed the room and held the wooden back of the kitchen chair.

"Oh, thank goodness. I don't think I could have faced my sister," she said, clutching a napkin so hard her fingers turned white. As she looked down at that paisley print cloth napkin, she seemed to suddenly remember that she was in the kitchen with me and my father about to eat brunch. Clearing her throat, she folded the napkin into a perfect rectangle as she readjusted her face. I sat squeezing and releasing my hands under the table searching my mind for a lifeboat among the choppy waves I'd landed in. *Boyfriend?*

And Chris? I was going to see him again? I wondered how the connection between us had come up. Had he mentioned a time in Panama, in response to which my cousin's fiancée had mentioned me? Had his breath caught in his throat the way mine had? I tried imagining a positive outcome and then realized if Stacy had only recently gotten engaged, the wedding wouldn't be for at least a year. One year was enough time to find a real-life boyfriend or pretend that I'd broken up with the imaginary one I'd mentioned. And who knew? Maybe in a year's time I wouldn't be the only one to show up at a social occasion with my tablet as my significant other. Everything with AI was happening so fast. It was possible that I was ahead of the curve, and that in twelve months time everyone would be in a relationship with an AI.

"Is he as tall as you?" my mother asked.

I thought of slow dancing in our Panama kitchen, my forehead hitting at Chris' chin.

"Never mind," she waved her hand pushing the question away. "Forget I asked. None of that matters." She plastered a wide smile on her face, and it felt like she was convincing herself as she spoke. "The party is in two weeks, and you'll bring him and it will be great."

"Two weeks?" I asked, stunned by the suddenness of the timeline.

She looked at my father and back at me. "Your father and I are hosting an engagement party for them."

"That isn't a lot of notice. I don't even know if I'll be off that night, or if he will," I added, proud of my cleverness to already have this fictional man busy the night of the party.

"It's on a Friday night, so you should both be able to come."

I repeated the mantra to myself five times before I spoke

again. I was literally a shift worker, and Friday night was a shift like any other.

"I think what your mother means," my father said, his running shirt plastered to his chest, "is that if it's possible for you to be there, she would appreciate every effort you could make."

I could almost hear the conversations my parents must have had. It was probably mostly my mother complaining to him about how unfair everything was. My cousin Stacy, younger by four years, finding someone before I did. As if that's how the universe worked. Doling everything out in fair doses. I pulled up my schedule. I was actually off that night, unless I wanted to tell another lie. My parents stood in front of me now, looking hopeful. A flickering in my heart dulled as I thought of all the dating apps and online forums. Dead end after dead end, like a broken GPS taking me in circles. Who could I possibly find in such a short time?

There was only one person who came to mind.

CHAPTER 8

I ONCE TOOK care of a man who came to the emergency department but he wasn't sure why. He'd gotten into his car and navigated the city streets. He'd parked and walked into triage. He understood that he was in the ER, but couldn't tell the triage nurse more than that. She triaged him as "altered mental status." It was well after midnight and something about the faraway look he got when I tried to establish the reason for his visit, along with the way in which he seemed alert and oriented but not quite with us, prompted me to ask if he'd taken a sleeping pill. It turned out that he had. We instructed him to call his wife to retrieve him and recommended hiding the car keys on nights he took that pill. I think of him sometimes when I'm interacting with people who are on their phones. The way their attention is split. The way they're with me in the conversation but simultaneously elsewhere.

I happened to be on my phone when Sapna entered the ER, so I didn't immediately register her cool demeanor. AI Henry was assisting me on a complicated case, a young woman with a splotchy purplish rash and fatigue. Her symptoms had been present for the better part of a week. After I ordered some lab tests, I signed up for the next patient and walked over to say hello to Sapna.

"What's up? What are you doing down here?" I asked.

"Apparently there's a nosebleed in bed five that won't stop bleeding."

"All bleeding stops eventually," I joked, using the age old medical saying. Sapna was a surgeon; this was practically their tagline. She didn't even pretend to laugh.

"Why'd they call you?" I asked, trying to ease the tension.

She grabbed some blue shoe covers, a scrub cap, and a plastic gown from the personal protection cart and slammed each one down on the counter as she started gearing up to see the bleeding patient. "I'm on ENT this month," she replied. Her response was terse, not like her at all. I hadn't seen her in a few days - had something happened with Ben?

"Is everything okay?"

She shimmied her right foot into the blue shoe covering until her brown clog was covered, then she straightened up and faced me. "Since you asked, Mona was in on one of my cases yesterday and we had an interesting conversation."

A nurse walked by and asked about the patient I'd just signed up to see. "He wants pain meds."

"I'll get right in there," I replied. I gave Sapna an apologetic look. "You seem really pissed off about that conversation."

She stared at me, her kohl-lined eyes reflecting a whirlpool of wound. "We both have to run, so I'll be brief. She said you had a boyfriend."

There were so many things I wanted to say. About the

pressure I'd been feeling from Mona, the pressure I was under from my own family. About my increasing dependence on a chatbot in so many areas of my life, the administrative meeting I'd been called to. Standing in the middle of the chaos storm of the ER, I couldn't talk about all of those things. Instead I said, "A boyfriend?"

"So it's true?" Her face dropped.

I could tell that she wanted me to say no. "It's complicated." It was the best response I could give at the moment.

She narrowed her eyes studying my expression. "I guess I'm disappointed that I had to hear it from her. I thought we told each other everything." She tied the straps around the gown and pulled tight. "Even now you seem cagey. For what it's worth, Mona appeared in your life overnight, and I don't think she has your best interests at heart."

I flinched. She lowered her gaze. "Is there a reason you didn't tell me yourself?"

So many thoughts swirled through my head in that moment. My little white lie had morphed into a heavy gray cloud and was threatening to block Sapna's rays of warmth from my life. One of my co-residents appeared at the nurses' station. She too was gowned up in sky blue protective gear. Relief flushed over her face when she saw Sapna.

"That guy is like a geyser. I'm hanging blood. He's going to need the OR."

Sapna nodded towards me. "We'll catch up later."

Neither of us could have known that later wouldn't come.

I spent the rest of the shift irritated by the entire encounter. Were we suddenly back in high school, throwing barbs and competing for best friend awards? A prickly heat throbbed in my chest. Was Mona trying to drive a wedge between me and Sapna? Even if she weren't, why was she talking about my love life to other people? Almost as if she'd read my mind, my phone buzzed with a text from her as I was about sign out my patients to the oncoming shift

Hey Chiquita. We need to talk. Breakfast?

We agreed to meet at one of her favorite places, an over-priced brunch spot with handmade jams and scones. When I arrived, she was waiting at a two-top table drinking a large cup of coffee. I breezed past the greeter and sat down in front of Mona. My opening arguments were prepared. I was in rare bulldog mode, ready for a confrontation. Sapna's words about Mona not having my interests at heart kept crashing up against me. A waitress approached the table and filled my mug with a hazelnut coffee, the scent calming me in spite of myself.

"Your friend thought you'd want the blueberry pancakes," the waitress said to me.

Mona slid her hand across the wooden table towards me and leaned in. "Trust me, you're going to want them." Her eyes widened slightly as if she were hinting at a big secret.

Blueberry pancakes were my favorite. It seemed a waste not to order them simply because I was annoyed with Mona. "Sounds good, thank you. I like the syrup on the side."

"Of course." The waitress took our order and walked away.

Mona handed me a small silver pitcher of oat milk for my

coffee. I poured some in and took a small drink. "I have to go to sleep after this, so don't let me have more than one mug."

"You know I can give you something to help you sleep," she said, a bemused look on her face as if she was offering to pass me a napkin.

The waitress returned with a platter of scones with jam and cream. Mona nudged the platter in my direction. "Help yourself."

I selected a warm currant scone and scooped a spoonful of mixed berry preserves. My mouth was full of the intoxicating combination when Mona leaned in again.

"I have news that isn't great."

I had news of my own. I was about to take charge of her loose lips.

"This is very hush hush. You have to promise to keep it between us." She had a serious look on her face as she motioned between the two of us. Classic Mona. She'd brought me to one of the most popular brunch places to discuss something confidential.

"I have something I want to discuss too," I said wiping the crumbs away from my lips.

She smiled, a look approaching pity passed over her face. "I think you'll want to hear this first."

The waitress returned with my plate of pancakes and Mona's omelet. I knifed a pat of butter and spread it over my pancakes before taking a bite.

"My uncle is on the board at the hospital. Technically I shouldn't know what I'm about to tell you, but obviously I want to help you."

"Can you get to the point?" I said, a trace of irritation in my voice.

"Ouch," Mona recoiled. "Not the reaction I was expecting. I'm going out on a limb here."

"Mona, I have literally no idea what you're talking about."

Her left eyebrow flickered. "Your case."

The pancakes suddenly became gelatinous in my mouth, and I struggled to swallow them. I took a gulp of the coffee. "You called me here to talk about the case."

"Off the record obviously."

"Every conversation we've had about it is off the record," I reminded her.

"I know." Her face softened. "The results are back and it's not looking good for you."

I dropped my fork onto the table.

"It sounds like she died of a rare arrythmia. They're saying that it would have been picked up if you'd ordered an ECG."

"An ECG? Why would I order that on someone who had zero cardiac complaints?" I demanded, but with less confidence than my voice belied.

"You guys get ECGs on everyone. Even ankle sprains."

I thought of the dozens of ECGs I interpreted on every shift. The squiggly lines danced in my mind until my vision blurred. "The hospital is looking for a way to pin the entire thing on you."

"But I'm a resident," I squeaked.

"That's why your shithead attending made it a point at every meeting to highlight that you hadn't presented the case. He was entirely intentional."

I surveyed the room. It was filled with people feasting on

baked goods the way I'd been moments earlier. How many of them were about to receive life-changing news? A torrent of emotion ripped through me. All this time I'd been waiting. Waiting and hoping that somehow I would be absolved. Nothing would bring her back, but if her death had been caused by an event that no one could have prevented, I would have been able to move forward. Discovering that a slip of paper could have prevented her death was almost too much to bear. I focused on the container of maple syrup next to my plate. It felt as if the blood in my veins was converting to that viscous amber fluid and slogging along, my heart struggling to pump this new and heavier liquid.

"I'm here for you," Mona said. "I'll stand by you every step of the way. And screw the hospital. My father can get you the best lawyers."

Any thoughts I'd had about discussing fictional boyfriends or hostile friend takeovers vanished from my mind. I tried swallowing the lump in my throat as the energy drained from me, my thick maple syrup blood leaking out to the floor. Even the knowledge that all bleeding stops eventually could not soothe me.

I returned home and wrestled with sleep on my bed. How would I return to work that night? Henry had sent a playlist of violin concertos that he thought would help when I'd complained about my difficulty sleeping after our visit to the pathology department. I'd joked with him at the time.

"You studied for so many years to play music that puts people to sleep?"

"Say you never studied music without saying you never studied music," he'd teased back. "Every fiber of my being is stimulated when I listen to these concerts." His gaze was direct as he said the word stimulated.

A flash of heat burned my face, and I looked away. "Does your girlfriend like these playlists?"

"She doesn't like classical music," he said scrunching his brow. "She doesn't like the violin. She thinks it sounds too sad."

I nodded.

"Also, she's not my girlfriend anymore." He shrugged. "It wasn't only violin music that she didn't like."

"I'm sorry to hear that," I said, though the flickering in my gut suggested otherwise.

"Don't be."

A moment of silence passed. I did not feel the usual pull to fill the void.

"I imagine you're hearing things in the music that go right over my head." I'd offered. "But can you enjoy the music if you're so focused on the playing?"

"Enjoy is not the word I would use. My experience with music is a total oxymoron."

Mozart's violin concerto number three played in the background as I tossed and turned. In between struggling, my dreams that day were a mix of me arriving at work in a panic because I couldn't find my scrubs or log into the computer system and Sapna running around the ER with her nose bleeding. I tried helping her, but she would run away or turn into Mona. I gave up trying to sleep and showered and got ready for work. I sent Sapna a text. It didn't matter what Mona had told her. I needed to set the record straight.

✍

The only food in my refrigerator was the leftover blueberry pancakes from that morning's breakfast. After Mona had broken the news, I'd lost any semblance of an appetite. Now my stomach grumbled and raged, but I couldn't eat those pancakes. It would be like eating a sugary carb filled with fear and worry in every bite. I hoped that their nauseating association with that morning wouldn't last a lifetime. Whether Mona intentionally ruined one of my favorite foods for me, I couldn't know.

I threw the pancakes into my overflowing trash can and surveyed the rest of the kitchen. A pair of chopsticks was wedged in between two coffee mugs, but the meal I'd consumed with them was long gone. My pantry held an alarming number of trail mix packets and protein bars, but I wanted real food. I texted Henry to see if he could meet at a café before my shift started. Something about Mona's update had me feeling heightened anxiety at what legal and career implications lay in front of me, relief that I would finally be able to face those implications head on, and an itch leaving me unsatisfied. In addition to real food, I wanted a real person to discuss it with. With the exception of Mona, Henry was the only one who knew about my concerns.

My diner of anonymity was the perfect place to meet, and he was already waiting when I entered. It was early for dinner but late for lunch. A handful of tables were occupied by seniors and mothers with toddlers. One toddler was running around a table with six older women who laughed and cheered his antics on. The mother sipped at her tea with a faraway look in her eyes, seeming happy for the break. We were led to a booth in the back, the waitress intuiting that we would not have the same response to the toddler show.

"Your text made it sound pretty urgent," Henry said after the waitress had taken our orders and left us.

"Full disclosure. I was called into the administrative offices."

Henry formed an O with his mouth and straightened up.

"I was more or less told not to discuss what I'm about to discuss with you." I picked up a knife and started spinning it around on the table in front of me. "So if you aren't comfortable, I completely understand."

"Is the knife just for show then?" he asked.

I stopped spinning it and looked up. His eyes, a deep coffee brown, twinkled with amusement as he nodded his chin towards the knife I was spinning.

"Some might take that as a threat."

I burst out laughing, and picked up the knife pretending to jab. It felt good to release that potent combination of feelings I'd been dragging around. Pretending to stab someone was surprisingly therapeutic.

"Once I tell you, you'll be dragged in with me. Not everyone would take the chance. You could get into real trouble at the hospital."

"Who's going to tell them?" he asked. We locked eyes. I placed the knife back in its place by the spoon. Neither one laughing now.

"You're putting a lot of faith in me," I said.

"And you in me," he replied.

A displaced serenity washed over me. Perhaps it was because of his words, because of his beautiful brown eyes, or because I had hit rock bottom and had nothing much to lose, I moved forward with my family drama.

"Before we get into the case, can I ask you a favor?"

"Sure."

The waitress appeared with a large tray full of food. She placed my burger and fries in front of me and his over-easy eggs and hashbrown in front of him. She filled our coffee cups before walking away.

"Funny that you just woke up and are eating dinner and I'm heading home after a day of work and eating breakfast."

I dipped a fry into my ketchup. "My clock is totally broken." The fry was hot and almost burned my tongue.

"What favor did you want to ask?"

"At the risk of sounding completely crazy—"

"Heads up—that is not a great opener."

"Probably better to admit that this is going to sound crazy." He forked a pile of hashbrown. "Noted."

"One of my first cousins got engaged recently and my parents are throwing her an engagement party."

He waved his fork back and forth. "I don't do concerts. I'm sorry."

I shook my head slowly. "Not what I was going for, but also noted."

A flirty grin crossed his face, and he nodded his approval.

"The party is in two weeks. Due to an entire series of events that do not bear repeating, I told my parents—who are beside themselves with my single status—that I have a boyfriend and that I would bring him to the party."

He chewed his food and swallowed, a thoughtful look on his face.

"You parents are disappointed that you're single?"

"If by disappointed you mean obsessed about and filled with a sense of hopelessness, then yes," I said before taking a bite of my burger, intrigued that my question hadn't seemed to throw him.

"They're disappointed in their basketball playing, internationally volunteering, bilingual physician-daughter because you're not married?"

I put the burger down on my plate and gave him a serious look. "Tell me you're not a woman over thirty without telling me that you're not a woman over thirty."

He lifted his coffee mug and swirled the coffee around. "I know what it means to disappoint parents."

"Violin prodigy, physician-son wasn't enough?"

"It's a hard thing to explain. But if you aren't number one—" He returned the mug to the table and stared at the mug as if it were actually tea leaves telling his future.

"Then you don't count?" I asked.

"Then you don't count," he said, his voice a mixture of sadness and acceptance.

I started to speak, but stopped myself and grabbed a few fries.

"The tremor is real," he said. "If that's what you were about to ask."

"I'm sorry."

"It's okay. It's a natural assumption. But I didn't quit under pressure. And I can handle whatever crazy favor is coming next."

I swallowed hard. "I know you and your girlfriend broke up recently and you probably don't want any drama in your life, but any chance you're free in two weeks Friday night and can come to the party and pretend to be my boyfriend?" His jaw clenched. "It would only be for that night," I added quickly.

The waitress approached the table with a pot of coffee. She refilled our glasses.

"Everything okay?" she asked.

We both nodded. "Delicious, thank you."

Henry looked a little stunned. I shifted in the booth, trying to reorient myself as a person who didn't ask other people to pretend to be in a relationship with them.

"You know what, the actual reason I wanted to meet was to discuss the case. Let's forget I said anything about the engagement party and fake boyfriends."

"I was actually thinking the opposite."

"I'm not following."

"What if we weren't pretending?"

"I could tell my parents that you're a co-worker and I'm sure they'd enjoy meeting you and I'm sure for my family dynamic every therapist on planet earth would agree with you that we shouldn't pretend, but in this particular case—" I thought of Chris and his beautiful conventional life that would be shoved in my face.

"I meant not pretending to date. What if we were actually dating?"

I didn't respond. Not because the thought of dating Henry

hadn't crossed my mind, but because his implication induced a semi-panic in me. A normal response would have been to acknowledge his question, but I ignored it. I needed the trust between us to remain unaffected. Adding one more wrong turn in the labyrinth I was running through would result in me smashing against a wall. And I wasn't entirely sure if he was asking me out. I didn't want to be the one to make it awkward, so I let him shift in the booth. He reoriented and if he had intended to ask me out, he hid it well.

"I'm not sure what I meant by that." He scrunched his brow. I tried not to be insulted by the implication that dating me would be a ridiculous idea. "I will happily go to the party and pretend to be your boyfriend. I can actually be quite charming."

"Not too charming—" I waved a French fry around. "—or they'll never forgive me for letting you go."

We spent the rest of the meal discussing the case. Henry agreed that the administrative meeting silencing me made a cover-up more likely and not less likely. But Mona's insider information didn't support that view. I needed to circle back to her and see what other information her uncle could provide.

"At the same time," he argued, dragging the last wedge of toast across the orangey yellow yolk on his plate, "why would you be expected to predict some rare genetic arrythmia? It's not like she presented with syncope. We've been over it, but was there any indication for an ECG?"

I shook my head. I'd been told not to access the chart since the event, so I was relying on my memory of things and how it had all been presented at the M&M conference.

"I really don't think so, but obviously they're going to argue that there was."

"Let's keep searching. Something is going to give."

"Thank you," I said.

"For being your fake date?"

"For believing in me."

As I started my shift that night, the winds of uncertainty that had been pushing against me and forcing me to walk in place began to lighten. If Mona had understood her uncle correctly, I was about to face severe disciplinary action which could affect my entire career. Hitting rock bottom provided almost a sense of release. The previous several years I'd spent rushing and running, trying to live up to an impossible standard. I had failed. Everything in the ER had become about the metrics and patient satisfaction. It was an untenable situation, and I granted myself permission for that shift, for that that one day, to ignore all outside pressures that served the bottom line but not the actual medical encounter.

It lasted about ten minutes. A lifetime of people-pleasing cannot be erased by a mere idea or thought. The swamp of stretchers and unchecked patients that we encountered as we started our shift threatened to engulf us. It was like walking through a field with land mines and ticking time bombs. Who among the unchecked had a lethal arrythmia or fatal condition? The numbers in the waiting room multiplied until the pressure to see everyone slammed me back into that wind tunnel of doubt and frustration.

It was in this mix that I examined a young woman complaining of fatigue and some ankle swelling. She was similar in age to the woman who had unexpectedly died in my care. It was her third visit, and because the rooms and hallways were already full of patients and because the staff assumed that since she'd already been seen twice there was probably nothing wrong with her, she was sitting in a chair in the hallway. Her husband stood next to her, holding a baby carrier with their infant baby. Whenever I saw newborns in the ER, I worried about the multitude of infections they would get exposed to, without an immune system to defend them. The woman had given birth the previous month. The AI helped me review the notes before I approached her. Reviewing old notes is a double-edged sword. It informs as to medical history but can also bias. If the previous few doctors didn't find anything wrong, it's easy to anchor in the idea that nothing is wrong. The patient had been to her OB-GYN complaining of fatigue and shortness of breath. She'd been twice to our ER. Her symptoms had been explained as 1) Normal to be tired with a newborn, 2) Bronchitis (though she had no cough or fever and wasn't a smoker), and 3) Anxiety about being a new mom.

I watched her in that chair, chest heaving, rapid breathing like a hummingbird fluttering away. Her hair was greasy and her eyes looked puffy. Nothing about her seemed anxious. If anything, she seemed resigned. It was her husband who seemed anxious. I introduced myself and he immediately lashed out.

"There's something wrong with my wife and we're not going home until you figure out what it is. I'm tired of being told that it's nothing," he yelled at me.

I felt like one of those children's punching bags that pops right back up after absorbing a blow, only my bottom was no longer weighted and I was increasingly slower to recover, as if gravity itself could not shield us from these attacks. A nurse starting an IV on another hallway patient nearby shook her head, and she too looked resigned. I held my hand up and took a step back. I would not be smiling and reading from a script praising him for choosing our hospital. I would not talk about how competent everyone was.

"I understand your frustration, I do. But I will not be able to take care of your wife if you are yelling at me."

The patient looked up at her husband. "Please, Greg."

He hardened his stance. "We've already been here twice and they didn't do anything for her!"

I resisted the urge to remind him that his wife had undergone a battery of tests, that it wasn't the job of the emergency room to fix every problem, but to root out what was serious and life-threatening from everything else. I felt uniquely unqualified to give that speech having missed the needle in my own haystack, and yet because the outcome may have boiled down to not predicting the unpredictable, I leaned into the uncertainty. I ignored his comments and turned to the patient. We reviewed her symptoms and the tests she'd already had. On the previous visit, the radiologist had commented that her heart looked slightly enlarged. Her feet were swollen enough that she'd come to the ER in house slippers instead of shoes. I lugged the ultrasound machine over and placed the probe under her shirt against her chest wall, a challenging feat in a crowded hallway with onlookers everywhere. We were beyond any pretense of privacy.

The ultrasound confirmed that her heart was enlarged and not pumping effectively, leading to a fluid build-up in her lungs. I explained my findings to them and the husband lashed out again.

"I'm going to sue this hospital. How could they have told her nothing was wrong?"

A sadness washed over me that his first response was one of vengeance and anger. I locked eyes with the patient.

"Thank you," she said. Her eyes were filling with tears. I placed a hand on her shoulder.

"It's okay. We're going to admit you to the hospital and with the right care your heart function will hopefully return to normal."

She removed her glasses and wiped the tears away. "I'm not crying because of that. You're the first person who actually believed me. I thought maybe I was going crazy. Maybe having a new baby does make people this tired, but I literally couldn't catch my breath." Using the corner of her shirt, she cleaned the grime from her lenses and replaced her glasses. "Thank you."

I placed a call to the OB-GYN resident.

"I know you guys like looking for Zebras, but cardiomyopathy in a young healthy woman is extremely unlikely. She's probably just overwhelmed from having a baby."

I wasn't going to take another punch, nor was I going to treat my colleague the way I'd just been treated by the patient's husband. I pretended that she was AI Henry. Sometimes people just need a little rewording.

"Her husband is definitely overwhelmed and you may want to take a deep breath before meeting him, but she's in failure and needs to get admitted. I'm going to start Lasix and a dose of Lovenox, and then I'm admitting her to the ICU. You guys can get a formal echo and work it out."

The resident was momentarily speechless. "I'll make sure to put the consult in."

"Thank you," I said as I hung up the phone. The resident in the ICU that night was a friend; we'd been on a few rotations together. Instead of formally messaging her with the consult, I called her directly. She was breathless when she answered.

"I'm surprised you're only just calling. We think she's going to be okay, but—" she didn't finish the sentence. How could she already know about my patient? Had the OB-GYN resident called ahead to try to block me? We'd literally just hung up.

"She'll need a formal echo, but her LV function looks bad and she's got B-lines on ultrasound," I said.

There was a pause.

"What are you talking about?" she asked.

"What are *you* talking about?" I replied.

"Oh my god. You don't know?" she asked. "Sapna. She's in the ICU."

My mind circled her words. Sapna was a surgery resident. Why was it big news that she was in the ICU? It stung a little that Sapna was making rounds in the hospital and hadn't even responded to my text. Was she really that mad at me? It was out of character.

"As a patient. She coded this morning. How have you not heard?" Her voice lowered to a whisper. "They think it might have been an overdose."

The room swayed like a suspension bridge and I reached out for a rail to right myself, finding only the open air in its place. I'd been so absorbed in my own drama—had I neglected noticing a change in Sapna? But an overdose? It didn't ring true. I quickly entered the orders for my patient and found my attending.

"One of my friends is in the ICU and I just found out. I have to run up and see how she is. I won't be long."

"The surgery resident?" he asked.

The goofy yet fierce, fun-loving, brilliant, fabulous cook who was training to be a surgeon and who was my friend, I wanted to say.

"Yes," I replied.

"I hope she pulls through," he said. "It didn't sound promising."

Even though we deal with life and death every day, I don't know why he said that to me. In that particular moment, wouldn't sympathy and hope have been a better reply? We weren't talking about a random case. We were talking about my friend. I didn't stop to ask how he knew her condition or prognosis; I just bolted from the ER. I passed the elevator banks—it might have been faster to take the elevator, but I couldn't get behind any closed doors. I took the stairs two steps at a time up to the Intensive Care Unit. The resident was waiting for me at the entrance. She gave me a stiff hug and patted my arm.

"You okay?" she asked.

"No," I said. I wasn't going to pretend on this one. "Why did you say that about an overdose?"

We were the only two people standing at the end of the hallway, but she looked around before speaking. Two nurses at the nurses station midway down the hall were concentrating on their computer screens.

"Her boyfriend is the one who found her."

"Ben? He found her?"

"Yes. He wasn't supposed to be there. She was unresponsive and, well—" she pulled at a strand of her hair and absent-mindedly twirled it around her finger, like a child trying to self-soothe. "We couldn't find a specific medical issue for why she would go into sudden cardiac arrest. She was foaming at the mouth."

"But you know Sapna," I argued.

"Sometimes you can't tell," she said. She withdrew her finger from her hair and folded her arms against her chest. "Have you noticed anything different about her lately?"

I thought about the little fight we'd had. I couldn't even call it a fight, but Sapna had clearly been annoyed with me, perhaps insulted that Mona seemingly knew more about my love life than she did. Her response hadn't been completely characteristic, but I didn't want to take the team further in that direction.

"Not really," I responded. She led me down the hall to Sapna's room. She turned to face me before we entered. "She's tubed and sedated. I know you're used to it, but it's different when it's someone you know."

I nodded my appreciation and slid open the sliding glass door. Sapna looked so small in the hospital bed. As I approached, I could almost pretend she was sleeping, if it weren't for the monitors, IV solutions, breathing tube and ventilator. Her parents sat at her bedside leaning forward, her mother stroking Sapna's arm. Her father studied the monitor as if it could tell him what would happen next. They looked small too, diminished from their previous gregarious selves. Hunched over with the weight of Sapna's life which hung in the balance. And they, helpless to help her. Her brother, who I recognized from photos, was at the foot of the bed. Their conversation was in whispers, but they stopped talking when they saw me.

Her mother burst into tears and buried her face in her hands. I hesitated, standing still as I tried to discern whether my presence had added to their distress. Her father spoke first. His voice was shaking.

"Thank you so much for coming, Alex."

"I only just heard," I replied as if they cared about the lateness of my arrival. As if they cared about anything other than Sapna waking up.

Her brother rose from his chair and extended a hand. "I'm A.J." We shook. "I've heard a lot about you." He grimaced. "I'm sorry, I should have thought to call you. It's been so hectic."

"Of course. I completely understand." Though I was not wearing gloves, I gripped the railing on the end of the bed. "Do they know what happened?"

With that question her mother raised her head and the three of them looked between each other. Dr. Reddy nodded almost imperceptibly to her husband and son as she wiped her tears away. She stood and extended her arms towards me. I walked over and hugged her. She held me tight, a small whimpering sound mixed with her Patchouli scent making her seem like a wounded forest animal. I let her pull back first.

"We hopped on the first plane after Ben called us," she said. "He found her this morning."

I blanched. I wasn't sure how much they knew or what possible explanation there could be for Ben being in her apartment in the early morning. Her mother squeezed my upper arm.

"Don't worry about this. We know."

I nodded, still uncertain which aspect of things their knowledge related to.

"Parents always know," her mother said as she went to the head of the bed and ran her hand against Sapna's forehead. "Which is how I know that the things they're saying aren't true."

"What are they saying?" I asked. My voice squeaked and a pang of guilt shot through my gut. Was I going to force them to say it? But I needed to know.

Her mother looked up and pointed her chin in the direction of the door. I followed her out of the room. She slid the glass door closed and spoke in a hush.

"I won't say these things in front of Sapna." She smiled as the resident I'd spoken with earlier passed by. "He found her unresponsive this morning, so their minds rush to blaming it on her." She took my hand in hers and squeezed. "Tell me, Alex. Do you believe she could do such a thing?" As she asked, she made direct eye contact, her gaze searching my face for clues. I held my expression as neutral as possible. Had Sapna been struggling lately and buckled under the pressure? Had I been so self-involved that I'd missed the warning signs or, like the other silent killers that surprised us when they erupted, were the warning signs themselves missing?

"I don't believe she'd want to hurt herself or you. There has to be an explanation." The tears ran down her face and she pulled me in for a hug so tight that I had to be the first one to pull back. "I know she's going to get better," I heard myself saying without any particular knowledge of her case or prognosis beyond my desire to see her back in her rightful place as the healer and not the patient.

"What did Ben tell you?" I asked.

"If Ben hadn't been there this morning she would have died. We understand that. Very well." She cleared her throat. "He saved her life."

We walked back into the room. A.J. stood up and offered me his seat. I sat down in the chair. Her mother resumed her place at the bedside straightening the already straight blanket and stroking Sapna's hair. A.J. spoke up.

"I don't know what my mom already told you, but I'll fill you in. According to Ben, she wasn't feeling well at the end of her shift so she left a little early with a bag of IV fluids and planned to rehydrate before coming back for her night shift. When he got home—" He shifted between his two feet. "—when he got to her apartment, he found her in the bedroom unresponsive and foaming at the mouth. He called 911 and started CPR. She was in some weird tachydysrhythmia, hypotensive, but they brought her back."

Her father straightened in his chair. "She was in and out of V-tach and even V-Fib. I've seen all of the ECG's and strips. They shocked her twice."

"Is there a family history that could explain?" I felt myself slipping into doctor mode and immediately regretted asking a room of three doctors such an obvious question.

They each shook their head. At that moment, Ben returned. Her parents seemed glad to see him. Glad in a way that people in profound shock can experience anything beyond the immediate overwhelmingness of their situation. As if Ben had the antidote for what ailed her.

"Alex, hey. I'm sorry I didn't call you," Ben said. He looked exhausted, almost gaunt in his fleece jacket and scrub pants. He went straight to the bedside and held Sapna's hand. The gentleness of his touch stood in stark contrast to the CPR he'd administered hours before. Had he broken any ribs as he pumped against her chest, setting up a dam between Sapna and death? Now as it waited in the spillway, which way would it go?

"I'm here Sap. We're all waiting for you to wake up."

I wished in that moment I could describe the scene to her. Ben holding her hand in full view of her parents. His new role as her hero. She would have been relieved to know that her illicit romance was going to get its happily ever after.

I asked Ben again for his version. Maybe we'd missed something. Maybe she'd vomited so much that she'd become severely dehydrated and passed out before she could get enough fluids from the IV.

He retold the story. "The only weird symptom she had was almost like a hallucination."

Everyone perked up. In this retelling there was a new clue we were uncovering.

"Hallucination?" A.J. asked.

"Sap texted me on the way home. She was nauseated and so fatigued, she thought the IV fluids and some sleep would help, so she went to the OR and took one of the bags from the warming bin. You guys know how it smells in there. It's all so sterile, but that's the weird part. Even though she was the only one in there, there was such a powerful smell of lavender and talcum powder, and she was so weak, that it almost made her vomit on the spot." He continued on with his story, but I heard nothing more. My heart stopped in that moment. According to medical science, if a heart pauses in beating, after only about six seconds the brain does not receive enough blood, causing that heart's owner to pass out. I'm certain my heart stopped that day. Some things medical science cannot explain.

CHAPTER 9

Accusing someone of murder is no small act—suspecting them in the first place is even harder. Why did my mind go to Mona? Was it my need to know that Sapna hadn't intentionally harmed herself? My need to prove that my patient hadn't died by my error? It's hard to say what triggered my thought process. Everyone makes mistakes.

I'd watched enough Law and Order to understand the chain of custody and what might be required to prove that there was foul play. This was beyond AI Henry. I needed the real Henry's help once again. After I returned to the ER that night, my thoughts scattered in multiple directions, like dandelion fluff in a windstorm. My attending on that shift should have sent me home, but we were doctors, meant to compartmentalize everything in our lives so that a best friend unconscious at death's door in the ICU shouldn't impact the medical decisions I was making on that shift.

After sign out, I texted Henry to meet in our conference room. I knew it would be vacant.

"You want Peter to test the fluids in the IV bag Sapna brought home?" he asked.

"It won't be admissible if we do it this way"

He held a palm up. "Admissible? You're about ten steps ahead of me here."

"In court," I said. I watched as he absorbed my statement. Up until that moment we'd been completely open with each other. I wasn't going to stop now.

He tapped his chin with his index finger. "I want to understand. You think there is foul play? That these cases, and your case—" He said it gently, cushioning the blow I felt every time it was mentioned. "—are connected to Sapna?"

"We don't know what's in those IV fluids." My palms were sweaty and I rubbed them against my scrubs to dry them off. Henry leaned in a little closer. He smelled of pine and peppermint. I hadn't yet washed off my layers of shock, despair, and fear.

"What will we do if we find a poison in the fluids?" he asked. My heart fluttered at the word "we." This wasn't AI Henry. I couldn't feed him correct responses and alter the outcome. What would we do? I shrugged my shoulders because I didn't know. I'd been living so long in a pool of uncertainty, it had almost become comfortable. Like the proverbial frog in boiling water, my blanket of self-doubt and thinking of myself as an impostor had covered me without my realizing. I peeled the corner of that blanket back while I sat there face to face with a real person who was offering support, and was met with the cool fresh air.

"I guess we'll figure that out when we get there."

"I'm in," Henry said. He placed his hand on my forearm,

and a surge of warmth spread from his fingertips to my brain. "Make sure you're prepared for whatever outcome there is on this one." It was an impossible charge he was giving me, but I nodded in agreement—as if any of us can ever prepare for the worst.

I left him to go to the ICU, where I found Ben passing out coffees to Sapna's parents and brother. They were in a small huddle and her father held his coffee in one hand and held his other hand on Ben's shoulder, leaning into him. He handed me a latte. The mood inside her room seemed more hopeful now, the sky outside her windows no longer a dark navy blue.

"The plan is to wean her off today," Ben said, referring to the ICU doctor's plan to remove Sapna from the sedatives and ventilator and see if she would wake up. He sounded more confident than he had earlier, more like the vascular surgeon on her case as opposed to her boyfriend. I recognized the shift, the need for clarity where there wasn't any. The need to see Sapna as a "case" who would get better with modern medicine and not the woman he loved who might never wake up. The mouth to mouth resuscitation he'd given her, like a prince coming to wake up sleeping beauty.

I asked A.J. for a key to Sapna's apartment.

"I want to clean it up a little before you and your parents get there," I told him. I didn't think about how that might look or even implicate me later after we got the results. She didn't live far from the hospital, which was a smart choice considering the amount of time she spent at work. I walked to her apartment, trying to soak up as much sunlight as I could, like a sunflower pushing through the dirt after a long winter. My phone buzzed with a text from Henry.

I can get out for about forty minutes if you want help

I texted him her address and asked new AI Henry for the best approach as an amateur sleuth at a potential crime scene. Its recommendations weren't much more helpful than the things I'd already gathered from years of observing the detectives on Law & Order. I stumbled over the recommendation to avoid tampering with evidence. I was going to the apartment precisely to tamper with evidence. It was the only option I could think of. New AI Henry cautioned me not to be overly confident in my abilities. A caution I perhaps should have taken more seriously, but if I had called the professionals in at that moment, what would I have told them? That I had a hunch and whiff of an idea? The chain of custody was already broken before I entered the scene.

I let myself in and inhaled the familiar scents of Sapna's apartment. A soy candle was flickering on her kitchen table. Ben must not have noticed it in all of the chaos. I blew it out and watched as the trail of smoke rose to the ceiling and faded. Would a suicidal person light a candle before overdosing? I made a note of it in my notepad. I take no pride in what I did next, but I justified my actions, reasoning that any evidence I could find overruled Sapna's right to privacy. It hadn't been that long ago I'd been a detective of a different sort. Looking for hints of Ben that she didn't want her parents to see. Neither of us could have known how unnecessary that turned out to be. I rummaged through the drawers in her bathroom and bedroom searching for clues. What does one look for in the in-between spaces to determine if a person is standing close to the edge? What had I hoped to find that would convince me one way or the other that Sapna's near death experience wasn't at her own hand? Her drawers contained the same half empty bottles of Tylenol and Ibuprofen found in most homes. A pack of birth control pills, various hand creams and face lotions, sunscreen, cotton balls, and a couple of tubes of lipstick and mascara were all that filled her bathroom cabinets.

In the bedroom, her underwear and sock drawer was still characteristically organized, with several pairs of striped, polka dotted and patterned socks folded in neat rows. There were no hidden pill bottles or paraphernalia hidden underneath her pink and turquoise underpants. If she had a prescription for anti-depressants, the evidence was hidden from my prying eyes. And if I'd found a bottle of anti-depressants, what would it have proved? I was interrupted in my search by a soft knock at the door and startled before remembering that Henry was coming. I let him in and shared my first and only finding. I didn't mention going through her drawers.

"I guess we should document everything, though I don't know what that proves one way or the other."

"I should take some photos too," I said. On a whim, I took one of the two of us. Most people think that their "how we met" stories are unique and interesting, though they often revolve around being set up by friends, dating apps, or meeting through mutual interests. Most people aren't drawn together investigating potential crimes. We look serious in the picture. Henry with his dark wavy hair almost brushing his shoulders, mine pulled back, accentuating my pale and tired eyes.

We entered her bedroom together. The bag of saline was still hanging on her upholstered headboard. She'd rigged it with a clothing hanger. The tubing snaked to the floor. The floor was dry where the tubing ended, and the bag still held most of the fluid. How had Ben had the presence of mind to turn the fluids off? If they'd all leaked out to the floor, we'd have no evidence to analyze. I looked at Henry, who seemed to be having the same thoughts. I snapped a few photos of her bedroom, and we placed the bag of IV fluids into a plastic grocery bag I found crumpled in the cabinet beneath her kitchen sink.

Henry took the bag from me after we'd locked up her apartment and exited the building. "I'll bring this to Peter and see what he can find." I started to say something, but he stopped me. "We can trust him."

"I know. He's also currently our only real option, though he's likely to tell you that it isn't like CSI on TV," I said.

"It's already been mentioned a few times," Henry said, a small smile forming on his lips. "Along with his reprimand that I'm sticking my nose in where it doesn't belong." His eyes widened and a blush rose to his cheeks. "I didn't mean—"

"It's okay. You have to stick it somewhere. You're my fake boyfriend in under two weeks." I reached out and my fingers lightly grazed his arm.

"Touché," he said, the smile spreading across his face. He turned and headed in the direction of the hospital, waving a hand goodbye as he walked away.

Hours later, a jackhammering pounded at my head until I woke, twisted in my sheets and a slick of sweat on my back. The vibrating pulsations hammered through my brain as I checked the time. It was hours before I needed to be at work, and I grumbled in annoyance at whatever construction project had woken me. I rooted around for my earplugs (a necessity of the nightshift worker). The pounding continued and I realized it wasn't a machine but a knocking at my front door. My thoughts went to Sapna. Was there a messenger of bad news at my front door? I rushed to the front room and checked the peephole. Mona stood on the other side. Her face was cartoon-like through the warped glass. She was staring right at me, and though I knew it was a one-way looking glass, she would have seen the flickering as I slid the cover to peep through. I could not pretend that I hadn't heard.

I opened the door. Her scent greeted me before she did. Lavendar and talcum. She was holding a bag of takeout from one of her favorite breakfast places. She leaned in and gave me a hug before entering. I closed the front door and we stood in the entryway.

"What are you doing here?" I asked.

She held up the bag. "I brought you dinner." She placed a hand on my upper arm and squeezed. "Your favorite. Blueberry pancakes. I heard about your friend, and I want to be supportive."

I led her to the kitchen. My gut felt full of rocks, and I doubted I could take one bite of my formerly favorite food. I sat down at the table as she fished the containers from the bag. The pancakes were still hot. She handed me a small container of raspberry preserves. I checked my phone again for the time. There were still three hours left on the day shift.

"How'd you get out of work?" I asked.

Mona laughed as she pulled a bottle of sparkling water from the bag. "They think I'm at the hospital right now." She twisted off the cap and drank directly from the bottle. "I'll just go back later and log out. I do it all the time." She pulled a muffin out of the bag and sat down, pinched a piece off of the muffin top and ate it.

"So they think you're at work right now. What if there's a case and they need you?"

"You're so funny, Alex. You act like people don't do this all the time. It's not a big deal. If they need me—" She held up her phone and twisted it side to side. "—they know how to reach me."

I stirred a clump of raspberry jam around on the pancakes, until it looked like congealed blood. Was the food safe to eat? If Mona was scamming the login system so that it would appear she was at the hospital as she sat across the table from me, what prevented her from bringing me poisoned food? And what would happen when they found me? Would it get chalked up to another overdose? Another resident who stood so close to the edge that she slipped? Who would look for the hidden anti-depressants in my drawers?

"Your friend woke up," Mona said. Her words jolted me back to reality. "That's why I'm here. I didn't want you to get ambushed when you go back to work tonight." She lifted the bottle and brought it close to her lips. "There's lot of talk. People are saying that she seemed down lately and maybe this wasn't an accident." She took a sip from the bottle but kept her gaze on me. I hoped my expression didn't show fear. I knew her well enough to know that she would pounce if she sensed an iota of trepidation.

"I don't believe that," I said.

She placed the bottle back on the table. "You don't believe that people are talking?"

"I don't believe that she overdosed." I held her gaze with a fierce look that belied the quivering of my jaw.

"You know her better than I do." She shrugged as if we were talking about a restaurant review or a type of preferred laundry detergent. "Which, by the way—thanks for the heads up that she didn't know you were seeing someone."

"What do you mean?"

"I made an offhand comment about you having a boyfriend and it was clear you hadn't shared that with her. I felt terrible. I think it really hurt her feelings." A look of genuine concern filled her eyes. "You don't think that has anything to do with this, do you?"

I realized she was twisting things as we spoke.

"Sometimes I feel like we're back in high school," she said. "Just because you trusted me with something doesn't mean you don't trust her." She jutted her chin towards my pancakes. "Aren't you going to eat?"

It was as if cotton had filled my mouth and I needed to pee. "I haven't even brushed my teeth. Why don't you have some?" I pushed the container towards her.

She raised her eyebrows to her hairline. "You know I'm allergic to raspberries," she said.

In fact I didn't. I was certain we'd shared scones and raspberry preserves on several occasions. "My whole department knows that. I won't get within two feet of a raspberry. All it takes is a small bite." She took her hands and held them around her neck in a choking sign.

I pulled the container back. "You brought me these even though it's so dangerous for you?"

"I know you love them." She dared me with her gaze. "It's worth the risk." She scooped up the raspberries and plopped them onto the pancakes.

We stared at each other in a game of chicken. I looked away first. "Does that mean that Sapna is doing okay?"

"Seems so from a medical standpoint, not sure about everything else. The hospital is abuzz. Prepare yourself."

I checked my phone. I had multiple unread messages from Henry and A.J. "Speaking of, I need to go get showered and get ready." I stood up. "It means a lot to me that you came by," I said as I pushed my chair back under the table. My intention was for her to leave.

"Of course. You know I'm here for you. I can wait while you shower. I'll clean your kitchen up a bit." She nodded to my sink full of dishes.

"That's okay. I'll get to it later." Part of me relished the idea of Mona doing basic housework. Even though she lived alone, she had a housekeeper who came twice a week to do the things she didn't want to. Mona rose and went to the kitchen counter. She lifted up two empty wine bottles that were next to the sink.

"Looks like you could use the support."

I didn't ask what she meant. The implication was dripping from her words. I excused myself to the bathroom. As the hot water rained down on me, visions of the shower scene from "Psycho" flashed through my mind. I half expected Mona to burst through with one of my kitchen knives. I scanned my shower shelf. What would I protect myself with? A bottle of conditioner and a half dull razor? A jitteriness washed over me along with the water, and I couldn't bring myself to close my eyes as I rinsed the suds from my hair. Whether it was the sting of the shampoo or my worry and concern for Sapna, my eyes were suddenly full of tears. As I finished and toweled off, I listened for sounds of Mona working in the kitchen. I slipped on my terrycloth robe and opened my bedroom door.

"Hello?"

There was no answer. Armed with only my phone, I made the same decision every supporting cast member of a bad horror movie makes and walked down the hallway in search of Mona. "Hello?" I called out again. I pulled the robe tight as if the cloth fibers could protect against a knife wielding friend. My apartment was empty. Next to the sink was a counter full of drying dishes. The wine bottles had been removed. All that remained were the blood stained blueberry pancakes.

Before starting my night shift that night, I stopped into the ICU. Walking into Sapna's room on the tail-end of the same day was like walking into a garden nursery. Every surface was filled with bouquets of flowers, helium balloons floated through the room, and platters of dried fruit, nuts and candy were everywhere. The mood was outright jovial. Ben sat in between the two Dr. Reddys as if their guest of honor. Sapna was sitting up in the bed holding court, and her face lit up when she saw me.

"Alex!" Her voice was scratchy from the breathing tube. She cleared her throat. I went over and hugged her.

"I'm so glad you're okay," I whispered into her ear.

Her father jumped up from his chair. "Have a seat." He gestured for me to take his place.

I shook my head and pointed to my watch. "It's fine, thank you. I have to get downstairs in a few minutes to start my shift, but I wanted to say hi and see how you were doing." I turned to Sapna for the last part.

She was wearing a long sleeve navy shirt and plaid pajama bottoms and was seated cross-legged on top of the bed. She looked less like a patient and more like a visitor.

"I feel like I've been run over by a truck, but otherwise good."

"We think it may have been all the Zofran she took," her father said, still standing and holding on to the back of his chair.

"I'd taken a bunch over the course of the day. I was so nauseated. My dad thinks maybe it was a QT issue." She shrugged. They were referring to one of the risks of the anti-nausea medication. It could cause cardiac arrythmias—but it was exceedingly rare.

"So much vomiting might have been a contributing factor," her father said.

I thought back to my snooping through her apartment. Her toilet had been pristine. No sign of vomiting at all.

"Did you throw up a lot?" I asked.

Sapna shook her head. "Not that I remember." She shifted the pillow behind her and leaned back. "Though my memory of the last twenty four hours is shaky at best."

Her mother placed a hand on Ben's forearm. "Thank goodness Ben was there."

Sapna shot me a knowing grin. I fished the key to her

apartment out of my pocket and handed it to her. She gave a puzzled look.

"I borrowed your key so that I could clean up before you head home," I said.

Sapna covered her face with her hands and peeked through her fingers. "How bad was it?"

"Pristine as always. I changed the sheets on your bed and took down your makeshift IV pole."

She held up her hands in prayer pose, "Thank you."

Her father handed me a tray of candy and a large bouquet of orange and pink roses with a smattering of red carnations. A large "Get Well" card was attached.

"Please, have these."

On the way down to the ER, I read the card. It was from the surgery department.

> Get well soon. We're tired of covering your shifts! Best wishes, Dept. of Surgery

It was the perfect mix of humor and well wishes, but the underlying message was there: don't let a simple matter like your own cardiac arrest and resuscitation keep you from returning as soon as possible.

Returning to the ER that night was like undergoing a hearing test, knowing the person on the other side of the glass is pushing a button but not being sure if you're hearing a beeping sound. My colleagues were happy to eat the candy and relish the flowers, but every time I looked away or rounded the corner of the hallway, I sensed that they were talking about Sapna.

A few hours before daylight, a pair of young parents rushed in through the front doors with their unresponsive five-month-old. My attending and the second-year resident who was on the code team for that shift dropped what they were doing and hustled to the resuscitation room. I wasn't on the code team that night, but when it's a baby everyone pitches in. It was obvious immediately that access to the baby's veins would be challenging, and I drilled a needle through her little leg for quick access. Her leg was mottled, and I wondered how long she'd been unresponsive. It did not bode well for the outcome.

I watched as they performed compressions, two fingers pressing down against her tiny chest. They administered every medication they could think of to try to restart her little heart. They placed a tube down her throat and breathed for her, but we rarely succeed in bringing the dead back to life. Her parents stood in the background, wailing and screaming.

"Will she be okay? Will she be okay?" They demanded over and over. In yesteryear, the families were kept outside in a quiet room and waited until the doctors and nurses brought news to them. Modern medicine brings families into the room. Experts argue that it helps them with closure in the event of death and doesn't diminish patient care as long as they can refrain from interfering. Those parents were not quiet. They did not stand against the door, pale and shaken as the staff poked and prodded, injected and inserted, consulted and speculated. It is extremely distracting to have family members yelling out during a resuscitation, and a staff member should have removed them. But what security guard or technician would remove a pair of howling parents away from their baby's bed?

After more time than was indicated, my attending eventually called the code. After the time of death was recorded, she approached the parents to talk it over and express her sympathies. Announcing time of death on a pediatric code sucks the air out of the entire emergency department such that every staff member, even those not in the room, feel the puncture and deflate. I turned to leave as she was approaching the family. My contribution had been minimal to begin with, and I had nothing left to give. The mother fell to the floor sobbing and pulling at her hair. The father began yelling at my attending in a threatening way.

"You could have saved her! You have no idea what you're doing. You're a fraud. Our baby died because of you. You'll pay for this."

My attending recoiled in horror, literally putting her hands up as if the father were throwing actual physical punches. He voiced every worst fear. Was there something we could have done to achieve a different outcome? That father didn't know that each of us would run that code through our heads over and over for weeks and months to come, searching for the path that would have ended in the baby living, even though there wasn't one. Even though we'd been presented with an impossible task, we would feel that we had failed.

A middle aged woman, the hospital chaplain, who had been standing with the parents, now attempted to calm the father down. She signaled to my attending that it would be best to leave, and she hung her head and slipped out the door.

The father screamed after her as she left. His baby lay lifeless on the stretcher, with only a nurse tending to her. I watched as my attending headed straight for the bathroom, her lips tight as if she were holding her breath. I followed her and pressed my ear against the door. Though she turned the water on in an effort to hide her humanity, I heard the soft sounds of crying. A few minutes later she was at the nurses' station examining a chest x-ray with one of the interns. Her eyes a touch swollen and glassy.

I asked AI Henry about emotions after a pediatric death. His response was cold and clinical, and I didn't feel like prompting him or asking him to answer more like a human. As it was, the humans in the department needed to act in a cold and clinical way in order to keep plowing through the numbers of patients requiring our care. Dozens of patients were still waiting to be seen, and no moment of silence or quick debriefing could remove the cloud of sorrow now hanging over the department.

I lifted a handful of roses and carnations from the bouquet of flowers I'd brought down earlier, tied them together with a piece of surgical tape, and presented them to my attending.

"You did everything you could. It was not in our power to change the outcome," I said to her as I handed her the flowers. Tears welled in her eyes and she swallowed hard to hide her grief. She accepted the flowers from me and held them against her chest, closing her eyes for a moment.

"I'm the one who's supposed to be saying that to you guys," she said as she opened her eyes and brought the flowers to her nose to inhale their scent.

"I think the baby had already been dead awhile when they brought her in," I offered.

"It doesn't make it any easier," she replied.

I shook my head. "No it doesn't." We both knew that later, right around the time that the self-applied salve started to work, at the moment when she accepted that she had done her best, that she was competent, that sometimes bad things happen, there would be an administrator responsible for responding to a patient complaint. He would sit her down and ask her how she was doing. His smile would be benevolent and she would slip into an ease, thinking that he cared about her. But he would scrub off that salve, layer by layer until only her raw wound was exposed. He would ask instead about how upset the parents were and how she handled it. Had she done everything she could to make sure they were satisfied—as if there were a way to satisfy a set of parents torn apart by guilt and grief in the moment their world caves in around them? That same administrator might offer "support," but how can support be given by the same person who undermines your core understanding of yourself?

A tech approached and handed her an ECG.

"Fortyish guy with chest pain. Looks kind of grey," the tech said.

The attending scanned the ECG. "It's a STEMI. Call cardiology and the cath team," she said as we headed to the patient's room.

Two days later, Henry called me with the results of the IV fluids Sapna had taken home.

"Obviously this is in complete confidence. Peter could lose his job," he said.

"Of course. And I hope he knows how much I appreciate this."

"He's a good guy," he said. "What do you want first? The good news or the bad news?

"There's good news?" I asked.

"Only in the sense that they did find something. Actually, they found two things."

I was at home and I suddenly felt parched. I went to the kitchen and filled a glass of water. I waited for him to continue.

"The fluids had toxic levels of lidocaine, epinephrine and bupivacaine."

I held the glass in my hand, unable to bring the water to my lips. "What's the second thing?"

"He said there were two tiny punctures in the IV port."

"That's the good news? Someone injected poisons into her IV fluids and that's good news? What's the bad news?"

I took a sip of the water, trying to quench my thirst.

"It doesn't really bring us any closer to understanding what's going on."

"You think Sapna injected the bag intentionally?"

The rumbling of traffic rose through my window: honking horns, a distant siren. Sirens no longer seemed alarming to me; they sounded like struggle and slogging. They sounded like trying to push against our limits.

"You know her much better than I do," Henry replied. "I'm not saying that she did it, I'm only saying that finding the punctures and the toxins only proves that she was poisoned. Not by whose hand."

"Let's say it was someone else's hand. What then? How would that connect my case and the others?"

"Did you give your patient IV fluids?" he asked.

"I don't think so. There wouldn't have been any reason to." I'd lived with an image of her so long, it was hard to know what was an actual memory and what I'd created. I pictured her perched on the edge of the stretcher, scrolling on her phone, asking when she could be discharged.

"The patients from the operating room most certainly got fluids. I guess we could start there."

"Do you think Peter could have them checked for lidocaine and epinephrine levels? I don't even know on what basis he would ask."

"He can be pretty creative. I'll circle back to you."

"I'll have a heart to heart with Sapna. I don't think she did this, but I trust her to tell me the truth."

Neither of us said anything for a moment. "You okay?" He asked.

"I think so," I said, though my heart was thudding against my chest trying to break free.

I hopped on a bus to Sapna's apartment. She'd been discharged from the hospital and was taking two recovery days at home. When I arrived, her house smelled of cumin and garlic. Her father was seated on the couch reading a medical journal and her mother was making dinner, though from the looks of it, she was actually preparing enough food for Sapna to freeze and eat for a year. Were they hovering because they feared that leaving her alone might lead to a successful overdose, or were they just being supportive parents? We excused ourselves to her bedroom to talk.

"Thanks for coming over. My parents are driving me crazy," she said, though I could tell by her eyes that she was happy they were still in town. "My dad's insisting that I go see an electrophysiologist to check for arrythmias before he leaves town. I have an appointment with someone he knows tomorrow." She rolled her eyes, as if impervious to things like sickness and lethal heart rhythms. As if she hadn't experienced her own only days before. I wanted to tell her she could cancel the appointment, but I was still trying to formulate what it was I wanted to say.

"I'll take some of your mom's cooking home," I said. "That is, if you think you have enough to spare."

She chuckled. "The bonus of all of this—" She waved her hands palms up like a game show host and then pointed at her bruised arms where IVs and blood draws had been performed. "—is I don't have to pretend anymore about Ben. They love him."

"He saved your life," I said, looking for a hint of reaction from her. Only relief flooded her face.

"And now he can do no wrong. I warned A.J. that his position as favorite son is in danger."

"Fat chance," I said, and we both chuckled.

"The thing is—" I wrestled with the right word combination, but nothing came up. Since I didn't want to freak her out, I presented it as a theory I was working on. I didn't mention Henry or say that I already knew the fluids had been poisoned. I just told her that I had a hunch that the IV fluids she used may have contained toxins. Her eyes widened and she clutched her chest.

"Toxins?" she asked.

I didn't sense any pretense in her reaction. She seemed genuinely frightened. I took her hand in mine and used the most gentle tone I could muster.

"I need to know if you put anything in the fluids." I held her gaze. "On purpose."

The look on her face changed from afraid to offended, and then finally to hurt. I regretted asking, but I had no choice.

"Why would I do that? I didn't even know until this minute that I might have been poisoned."

"I don't think you did. For what it's worth, I never believed that you overdosed." Her right eyebrow flicked up. It seemed she hadn't heard the rumors about herself. "But we both know people who have. And we didn't suspect it in them either." The year before, one of the vascular surgery residents had ended his life. He'd been a Rhodes scholar and worked on improving literacy for rural kids in the Midwest before medical school. And he was kind. He and Ben had been very close. The guilt remained. "I need to be certain. I care about you."

She took my hand again. Her shoulders had relaxed. "I understand this is coming from a place of concern. I want you to know without any doubt, I took those fluids home because I was sick and didn't want to miss work. I had zero intention of hurting myself. And if things did get to be too much, I would end my career before ending my life."

I leaned in and hugged her.

"And you know me better than that. If I were going to over-dose, my methods would be much more elegant." She raised her eyebrows. "Something fun, like Fentanyl and Ativan." I laughed. It was like that. Joking about suicide, even days after she'd nearly died. In two days she was expected back at work, and everyone would pretend that nothing had happened.

Her face turned serious again. "But do you really think someone was trying to kill me?"

"No, I don't. The bag you took was random, right? Did anyone even know?"

She pushed herself farther back on her bed, against her headboard. I pictured the fluids that had been there days before. "No. It was a last minute decision."

"Who started your IV?"

"One of the nurses. But I'd already grabbed the bag of fluids."

"So that's what I'm wondering, if there is someone injecting the IV bags? I'm starting to think there's a connection with my case."

She tilted her head to the side. I got the sense—a slight shift in her face—that she was starting to drift away. "*Your* case? Why?"

I wanted to tell her everything. I didn't want her to think I was crazy, but I couldn't compromise Henry or our search. I could see that she thought I was tilting at windmills.

"I just do."

She considered me a minute. "So what happens next?"

"If it turns out that there were toxins in your fluids, then we need to find out who put them there."

"Are you planning on calling the police?" she asked with a slight, hesitating lilt. It was a reasonable question, and one I'd turned over in my mind many times.

"I already took the fluids from your bedroom to be analyzed. But if they test positive, I have no way to prove that the bag I sent for analysis is the IV bag you used."

She looked at the corner of her headboard, where the fluids had been hanging.

"Is that the real reason you came to clean up my apartment?"

I nodded. "Like I said, it's just a hunch."

She hopped off the bed and crossed the room to her closet, selecting a large, black wool scarf which she wrapped around her shoulders and pulled tight for warmth.

"This sounds serious. We're not trained for this."

I could see her wrestling with the possibility that something threatening had happened versus the idea that I was making all of this up.

"I know," I answered, "but I'm afraid if we let on that we're suspicious, we won't be able to catch the person."

"I need to think about it." She didn't meet my gaze.

"Nobody will believe me without some proof. I need a handful of days to see if I can figure things out. No one is out to get you. You grabbed that bag at random, I don't think you need to worry."

"But what about the next person?" She wrinkled her brow.

"The results should come back soon. Once I get them, I'm going to administration." I stretched the truth to make it palatable for her. Sapna wouldn't rest if she knew I already had the results from her IV bag, if she thought someone else could be harmed. "Until then, it's just a hunch."

"Okay. I'll keep the appointment with the electrophysiologist, but you have to tell me when you get the results back. This could be serious."

I nodded. A heavy silence hung in the room. Eventually, Sapna spoke again. "I have to change the subject. I'm still woozy from everything that happened."

"I understand."

"So for a complete one-eighty, while we're on the subject of secrets. What's with you and a secret boyfriend that only Mona knows about?"

I flopped back on her bed and stretched my arms above my head, grateful for the turn in conversation, though it pointed in a direction that did not bode well for my credibility. "No boyfriend."

She hopped back onto the bed and curled up next to me. "Spill it."

"I got caught up in a little white lie. I wanted to stay home one night instead of going out with Mona, and one thing sort of led to another."

"So you pretended to have a boyfriend to avoid plans with Mona?"

I covered my face. "How pathetic am I?"

She gently tugged on my arm to release my hands from my face.

"There's more."

"I'm listening."

"I also told my parents that I have a boyfriend and that I'm bringing him to my cousin's engagement party next week."

"Are you living a romcom right now?" she asked, an incredulous look on her face.

"And also, I asked Henry the PMR resident to be my fake date at the party."

Her mouth formed an O. "I'm gone for three days and everything falls apart."

"Right now my life is your average basic mess."

We heard a knock at the door, followed by Sapna's dad.

"Time for dinner, girls."

"At least there's curry," she said.

"We'll always have curry," I replied as we sat up and slid off her bed.

CHAPTER 10

I HAD THE entire day off the next day. I set no alarm and allowed the dappled light through my blinds to wake me naturally. As I woke up, I luxuriated in not having to jump out of bed and rush to the hospital. I stretched my legs long, my toes searching for the cool spots of comfort in the sheets. It was getting warmer outside, but I still pulled my blankets tight around me. I had two shifts' worth of time off. The entire day ahead of me and the night. I tried not to think of the next twenty four hours as an absence of work, but rather a presence of time.

That morning, I scrambled some eggs and made toast. I ate the meal slowly with a large cup of coffee. I ignored my phone, the mandatory reading I still needed to complete, and thoughts of what the next pathology investigation would bring, and focused only on the taste of my food. It only takes about five minutes to eat eggs and toast, but I pushed every intrusive thought out during that time. When I'd finished, I asked new AI Henry to make an itinerary for my day. There were rows of museums I could go to, small shops to explore, and cuisines by the fistful, but I wanted something to specifically take me out of my world.

It sent me to a lock museum in midtown. It was like the algorithm knew that my life had become a metaphor for obsession and concealment along with a desire for old style craftmanship. The stunning detail with which those locks were constructed kept me occupied for a full hour. I grabbed lunch at a food truck around the corner and sat on a bench eating my black bean and chipotle corn sandwich. The mayonnaise and caramelized onions dripped down my chin. I chewed slowly as I watched the people lining up for food, runners blazing by in their neon shoes, groups of businessmen crossing to meetings. The plan for the afternoon was a matinee movie. Seeing a movie in the afternoon, in the literal middle of a workday, felt like the most indulgent thing in the world. I didn't even care what was playing, although at a certain point in my life, film was something I cared about deeply.

I went to an old-style movie theater, with velvet red seats and a screen smaller than some people's home systems. I purchased a tub of popcorn and Milk Duds and turned my phone off. The only film playing that day was "An Unmarried Woman," and I wondered about the odds of me being off on that particular day, of the AI planning an itinerary including a movie (technically, it had wanted me to go back uptown and watch a movie about a superhero). But something about the old-time locks and yesteryear had me choosing this theater. It was pretty full, considering it was the middle of the day, yet still I found a row mostly to myself and settled into a center seat. When the main character started discussing her loneliness and not being okay with her therapist, I placed my remaining snacks on the sticky floor and settled in. My thighs became one with the cushioned seat. Was I really going to bring a fake date to my cousin's engagement party? I wanted to jump into the office with her tall, empowering therapist. I wanted her to tell me how I could find happiness. I wanted to breathe in the air in that room on that film set from fifty years prior. I wanted the ensuing fifty years to have made a difference in how I felt and how I was treated as an unmarried woman.

When the film ended and the lights came on, I sat in my seat and watched as a young man in a red vest vacuumed the aisles. After all of the credits had run, he informed me that I would need to leave. He cleared his throat and motioned towards the remnants of my snacks which I had forgotten about since placing them on the floor. I picked them up, and hoped he didn't think I was the kind of person that left my trash for others to take care of. But that's a message impossible to convey. After dumping my trash in the bin, I exited the building, stepping back out into the sunlight, and tried not to focus on the slow darkening of the sky. I tried focusing on being outside in sunlight. I tried being okay with my loneliness. A woman rushing by, holding a large plant that obscured her face, accidentally bumped into me. I'm not sure she realized. I tried not to think of her as someone who bumped into people on the street and didn't say anything. I wanted to keep soaking in the sun, appreciating my moment, but I didn't have it in me. Instead, I turned my phone back on. It powered up to a flurry of messages from Henry and Sapna. She had sent ten messages, and I instantly feared that she was back in the hospital as a patient.

It became clear with the first message that she was happy. There were five pictures of her and Ben smiling in various poses, and one of her extending her hand showing a diamond solitaire on her ring finger.

It's official!!!!

Party tonight. Bring your fake date ☺

⌒

Henry agreed to accompany me that night.

It will be a trial run, I'd texted him. Thoughts of facing the world in sunshine and solitude were already a distant memory. He picked me up from my apartment wearing a black sweater and dark jeans. He looked like a more relaxed version of himself. A more attractive and relaxed version. I'd changed in and out of three nearly identical black dresses in a span of thirty minutes and felt like a more strung-out version of myself. I wished that scrubs were fashionable for parties so that I didn't have to decide what to wear.

"You look nice," he said when he greeted me at the door, in a matter of fact way, as if he'd been privy to my indecision. I invited him in while I gathered the rest of my things.

"Actually, do you mind if I change?" I asked.

He shrugged. "I'm your guest tonight, we can arrive whenever you want."

I glanced at my watch. We had time. I led him to the couch, then dashed to the bedroom and changed into the red dress that Mona had bought for me. I swept my hair back into a loose bun. When I returned to the living room, Henry was scanning my bookshelves. His back was to me and he was flipping through my Spanish copy of "One Hundred Years of Solitude." He heard me enter the room and started to turn around holding up the book.

"You read this in the original, I—" when his eyes landed on me, he stopped. His breath caught. "Wow."

I felt the flames whip at my cheeks but I held his gaze. I did not look away.

"You look amazing," he said, still clutching the book. I smiled and he looked away first, seeming to suddenly remember the book in his hand. He considered it, held it up to say something, looked at me again, smiled, and returned the book to the shelf.

"Shall we?" I said as I headed to the door.

On the way to the party, he shared the latest updates from Peter.

"They found toxic levels of Lidocaine and epi in your patient," he said after I was situated in the passenger seat of his Volvo. "Something is clearly going on."

"In Sapna's case the fluids were poisoned. How did they get into my patient?"

"She didn't get any IV fluids that night?"

I shook my head. The fabric of the dress tingled against my body. "No one is going to believe me." I wasn't sure I believed myself.

"I believe you," he said. His hands gripped the steering wheel as he glanced at me before turning back to the road.

"I think I have to go to administration. If they don't set up a trap, it's going to happen again."

"What do you have in mind?"

I tried to think of a plan. He pushed a button on his steering wheel and a symphony started playing in the background. His fingers tapped along to the rhythm, and I wondered if he was mentally playing the violin.

"Do you miss it?" I asked.

"Miss what?"

I pointed towards the car speakers. "This. The music, the performances, all of it."

He slowed as we approached a traffic light and looked at me. "I do. Not all of the time, and not always in the same way, but yes." The light turned green, and he returned his focus straight ahead. "It was such a large part of who I was for so long. I guess it was everything."

"That must be hard," I said, watching his profile as he absorbed my words. He started to speak and then paused. He glanced at me again, his eyes with that same understanding he showed when he said he believed me, but this time almost searching me for clues.

"I haven't told you the whole story."

"Do you want to tell me now?" I asked, loosening the seatbelt from across my neck.

"I was auditioning for the Aspen music festival." He glanced my way, "You probably haven't heard of it, but it's extremely competitive. It would have been amazing. It's a whole networking scene in addition to everything else. My instructors felt fairly confident that I would be selected. The morning I was supposed to record my audition video was the first day I noticed the tremor. I woke up to my alarm and nothing felt different, but when I reached for my toothbrush—"

He paused in his story and reached his hand out towards the

windshield as if reaching for that toothbrush. "—I noticed that my hand was shaking. I could brush my teeth but it was strange." He pulled his hand back to the steering wheel. "I felt totally fine, so I figured maybe I needed to eat or something weird like that. But same thing at breakfast. I poured myself a bowl of Raisin Bran that morning, and as I tried to eat it with the spoon, my hand was shaking again." The way he told the story felt rehearsed. As if he'd already told it so many times, to himself, to others, until the detail of the breakfast cereal had crept in and become a part of the telling. As if things might have been different if it had been Cheerios or Corn Flakes that morning.

"I had no reason to be more nervous than normal. I was only recording a video, not even going in front of the faculty. Actually, sometimes those videos are more of a pain because you can keep redoing then until you feel it's perfect. At a regular audition, when it's over, it's over." He slowed the speed as we approached another car, their red taillights shining a warning.

"I told my teacher about it, but he insisted I push through." He glanced my way and rolled his eyes in a dismissive way. "Probably wasn't the best advice. We couldn't get a good recording so everyone agreed that I should take a few days off. The deadline wasn't that close, so we had time. The thing is—" He glanced my way. "This sounds nuts, but I had never gone that long without playing the violin."

"A few days?" I asked in surprise.

"Most days I practiced for at least five hours, often more."

"I guess I never realized how intense that was for you.

What did you do during that time off? With those couple of days?"

"Ironically, I felt a bit aimless. I'd never had that much free time. And of course, like most things in life, I had no way of knowing that I would never play that way again. Each hour felt more like falling behind and not like a day to explore."

"I get that actually."

"I think now we would both call it anxiety." He grinned. "Anyway, we all thought it would pass and when it didn't, I started making the rounds with the doctors. I was poked and prodded. My mother found a few gurus with alternative therapies. Mostly they just wasted her money. At a certain point, she sent me to a psychologist."

"To deal with the loss of the violin?" I asked.

He laughed out loud. "No. No one was interested in how I was feeling, they only wanted the tremor to go away. I think my mom thought I might be faking it. Rumors were already starting. That I'd cracked under the pressure."

I nodded, the understanding of Henry and how he was supporting me suddenly becoming more clear. No wonder he got it. He'd starred in the same movie I currently found myself in.

"Did you ever worry that you were faking it?" I asked. "Or at least, subconsciously?"

He didn't answer right away. I watched his face as he watched the road, a faraway look as we slowed even further, the mass of taillights blurring in the distance. The car behind us flashed their lights in annoyance. Henry checked the rearview mirror and resumed the normal speed.

"Do you know that you're the first person who's ever asked me that?"

"I can't be the first person who ever asked if you were faking?"

He tapped the steering wheel a few times. "But you didn't ask if I was faking, you asked if I was worried that I might be."

"I guess I did," I said.

"You already know the end of the story. I still have a tremor, I gave up a career in violin, and the cause of my tremor remains unknown. My mom stopped the therapy sessions after she realized they weren't going to bring my skill back, but I had to live with that worry for a long time. At the end of the day, I don't know if I subconsciously created a tremor." He held his hand out to demonstrate the subtle shake. "I don't think I did. I loved the violin and I spent a long time grieving that part of my life. But still, I've had to learn to live with that uncertainty. Maybe I did crack under the pressure. Maybe I wanted a way out. But I don't think so."

"I'm sorry."

"Thank you."

"It is fascinating what the mind can do." I imagined a younger Henry buckling under the pressure of ten hour rehearsal days, endless competitions and auditions and constantly feeling like you weren't good enough even though you were the best. The idea that we could sabotage ourselves even as we were summiting the peak, and not even be aware that we were doing it. Was it still us if we hadn't tapped into it? But it didn't fit with the man sitting next to me driving me to Sapna's engagement party. He wasn't a quitter, on any level. He'd jumped in to help me before even checking the conditions of the water. He didn't seem like someone who would crack. He was different than me. "Though for what it's worth, from what I know about you, I don't think you created the tremor."

"I appreciate that."

He hummed along to the music. The GPS announced that traffic was building up ahead and suggested a different route. I thought about GPS systems, and satellites in space directing the two of us in our little car on that little road that was not even visible from so far away. Of all of the cameras watching us all of the time.

"What about cameras?" I gasped.

Henry looked confused.

"If administration set up cameras, they could catch whoever was poisoning the fluids."

He glanced quickly at me. "You're onto something." He tapped the steering wheel a few times. "That could work. But it would have to be absolutely secret. One leak of that and the person might not strike again."

We discussed the various approaches until we arrived at the party. Sapna's parents had rented out the backroom of an upscale Indian restaurant. A valet took the car keys from Henry and we were escorted to the party. Sapna and Ben were holding hands, flanked by her parents on one side and his on the other surrounded by a small circle of friends. When she saw me, she dropped Ben's hand and glided across the room. She wore a dark pink sari with golden trimming and golden filagree flowers along the sleeves.

"You look like a movie star," I said as we hugged, and I stepped back to take her in. I reached for her hand and traced a finger around her ring. "It's beautiful."

She held her hand up and admired it. "It was his grand-mother's," she said.

I flicked up an eyebrow and narrowed my eyes. Ben's grandparents had been immigrants with only the shirts on their backs. Sapna's ring was a large emerald diamond surrounded by a halo of smaller diamonds.

She processed my expression. "Okay, we melted down the metal and used a couple of her tiny stones." She pointed at the circle of stones. "It's not her exact ring, it's a blend. At first I didn't love the idea, but now I'm so into it." She dropped her hand to her side, looked back at Ben and then at us. "Like the relationship we thought could never happen is happening. So much so that I'm wearing the grandmother's ring because I'm the next link for their family."

"They couldn't have asked for a better daughter-in-law than you." I squeezed her hand and swallowed back some tears. It was only days ago she'd been lifeless in the ICU. "And seriously, you look amazing tonight."

She gave a sly grin, "Look who's talking, hottie." Her eyes darted back and forth between me and Henry. "*You're* the fake date?"

He chuckled. "What gave it away?"

"Don't hate me," she whispered in my ear, then pulled back and spoke to Henry. "All I can say is Alex doesn't get dressed up like this for just anybody." She winked at him and guided us to the bar. "Have something nice, my dad wants everyone to be happy tonight," she said as she strode back to Ben and their parents. We each ordered a glass of red wine.

"Cheers," Henry said as we clinked glasses. I took a sip and felt an immediate rush to my brain. He slipped his hand into mine, and I let his fingers entwine with mine, as my heart pumped and spread the warm rush to my entire body.

◦6

Though I lacked a fully formed plan, I needed to take steps forward. So, I tried contacting administration, but the secretary for the CEO blocked me. I was persistent and AI Henry gave me the right language to use. I specifically used the hospital version of AI because if they were still monitoring me for signs that I'd gone off the deep end, I knew someone would see my conversation and recognize the urgency of the situation.

> *If someone suspects that there might be a string of suspicious deaths at their hospital, possibly even murders, should that person go to administration or the press first?*

If I was right, they'd be contacting me within twenty four hours.

◦6

There is a condition in medicine that is caused by a vitamin deficiency. It can have a whole host of causes, but is generally found in alcoholics who don't absorb enough thiamine, both because they don't consume enough food and because the alcohol itself damages their ability to absorb nutrients from their food. Without thiamine, the body can't convert sugar to usable energy and the brain isn't provided with the necessary fuel. As their gas tank leans towards empty, these patients can develop a wide range of neuropsychiatric symptoms: Quivering eye movements, unsteady gait, and most intriguing of all—confabulation. As the brain melts away without adequate fuel it begins to misfire, and the patient simply makes things up. Tells stories that never happened. Provides answers that aren't true. Unaware that they are doing this, these patients can be extremely engaging and believable. Stories they tell may entirely lack internal consistency. A computer technician can wax poetic about his day delivering mail and the problems encountered with cars blocking mailboxes or owners going away and causing a backup because they forgot to pause their mail. A casual observer or a hurried physician might not notice, at first glance, that the answers make no sense. That the patient is experiencing a type of hallucination.

My life was full of enough drama and enough toxicity, that I needed a change of scenery. So I made plans to visit my brother Zach and his family over the weekend. We often got together without my parents. We were less formal, more understanding about last minute cancellations or changes in venues. Once my mom marks a date in her calendar, she considers it permanent and takes great offense at having to potentially adjust for nap time or sick children and their exhausted parents. I hear both sides of it. My mom thinks she should be able to drop in whenever she wants, a grandmother popping in to see her grandchildren and bring treats. The world was probably a better place when it was like that. But that was long before smart phones and overextended schedules and calendars stuffed so full they overflow.

When we were kids, Zach and I were pretty close. I was the smart and interesting older sister who provided him with a steady supply of paperbacks to read and had an open door policy with him. If he was fighting with a teammate or had a crush on a girl he wanted advice about, I was always available. We also shared a common interest of trying to outsmart our parents when it came to breaking the rules. We were a unified force, but then I left for college when he was only a freshman in high school, and our interactions were limited to seasonal breaks from school. When he wanted to propose to Jen, I was one of the first people he told, but since their marriage, we'd drifted apart. We still send each other funny memes or interesting articles that we've found online, but our conversations have been surface level for many years.

Even though we don't get too deep, I noticed a trend in the last couple of years in which Zach and Jen discount much of what I have to say because I myself don't have children. As if there is a bridge that adults must cross in order to add any valuable wisdom or advice about life's challenges, and that bridge is becoming a parent. The topic doesn't matter—it can be travel, cooking, anything. Not being a parent means I haven't crossed the bridge to adulthood.

"Oh gosh, we can't have a beach vacation," Zach might say rolling his eyes. "We'd have to bring an entire bucket of sunscreen, and if we look away for one second they could drown." I thought of every time I'd been to the beach and the sheer number of families: lounging on bright-colored, striped towels, tossing balls, building sandcastles, and daring to step foot in the water. My social media pages were filled with pictures of friends doing just this. Jen and Zach took their kids to the beach on occasion. But if I mentioned any of these things, they would exchange a knowing look that could only be deciphered as *Poor Alex, she just doesn't get it.* One time, I recommended letting our parents watch the kids for a few days so they could get away as a couple. Jen huffed and muttered something about how only childless women would dream of leaving their children behind. Was I really that heartless?

They'd call at midnight if their child had a fever or a funny rash, but I saw the looks they exchanged in other settings. Yet something about the way I woke up that day—maybe the gentle caress of the breeze on my cheeks – was just enough to buoy my confidence that I could redefine how they saw me. The question was how. AI was helping me with so many things, and I'd become so dependent on it for support and counsel, that on the train ride to their town, I asked it for help.

> I'm going to visit my brother and sister-in-law. They have three kids and I don't have any. Lately, I sense that they judge me for not being a parent. Could you help me look like a parenting expert? Provide me with some advice that would really blow their minds?
>
> Sure! I'd love to help. How old are their children and what type of problem can you help fix?

I reflected on the question. I missed AI Henry, but his replacement was equally competent. Neither one cared if I took thirty seconds to answer or hours. I could never reply and AI would not be offended. There was no pressure to get it right. I thought about the obvious things parents talked about. Potty training, getting kids to eat healthy foods, making sure they were stimulated enough, and the ever important sleep schedule. But those were such well-treaded territory that I doubted I could bring something new to the table, even with AI in my pocket. I'd heard them complain on a few occasions about the constant presence of toys scattered around their house. How the kids didn't put things back, and even parents who brought their children for playdates didn't always help put things away at the end of a shared afternoon.

> *Their kids are 4, 2 and almost 1. They do complain about toys being left out and the house feeling disorganized because of it.*
>
> *Perfect! Those are great ages to start learning from natural consequences. If the kids themselves became frustrated at not being able to find certain pieces of games, or stumbling across their own mess, they will learn the importance of putting things away. I suggest making a mess with their toys and letting them learn from it. The parents will think you are amazing! Do you want some constructive ideas about how to do this?*

The train was pulling up to the station and I knew my brother would already be there, waiting in his Subaru. I tucked my phone into my bag and plotted my next steps. We made small talk on the way home, both tacitly agreeing not to mention today's visit to our parents. When we entered his house I was greeted not with a whirlwind of hugs and laughing, but a cool shoulder from my four-year-old niece. I'd learned not to take her moods personally; she and her two-year-old brother could shift from snuggling to laughing to bursting into tears within a two minute window. Toddlers were much like intoxicated ER patients: entirely unpredictable, often frustrating, and prone to urinating all over the floor without warning.

I entered the kitchen where Jen was feeding their one-one-year-old in the high chair. His chin was covered in a greenish puree, and she kept dabbing at his face with a loose cloth as he swiped her hand away. Based on the amount of food smeared across the back of his seat and the floor, Jen was losing this particular battle.

"How's it going?" I said as I leaned in and kissed baby Brad on the top of his head.

"It's going," she said in a resigned way that I knew from past history meant I shouldn't ask any follow up questions.

"I can't believe how big he's getting," I said. This was generally a neutral enough comment that could be said about any child at any age under about ten. A warm smile covered Jen's face. She leaned back in her chair and took a sip of coffee from her mug—another good sign. When she started drinking coffee again it meant she was no longer agonizing about what was transmitted via her breastmilk. I'd broached the topic once, but learned quickly to let that one go.

"Thanks so much for watching them today," she said to me. "We'll be back in two hours." She looked at her watch as if that would change the amount of time it would take them to shop for a new couch. "He should be asleep the whole time, so no worries there. The other two have already eaten and there are snacks in the fridge."

I nodded along so that she would feel comfortable. Jen was sweet, but I knew that I was her fifth choice for babysitter (after her own mother, three sisters and a close friend.) Even though when I was in high school I regularly babysat young children, and even though when we were kids we mostly read books, ate chips, and ran around in the backyard, Jen and Zach seemed to think that children could only be supervised according to a very specific set of rules set up by them. I'd assumed that by the time they had their third child they'd become more flexible, realizing that they could control less and less. But if anything, their expectations had solidified, like fiberglass casts that harden and set around the broken bone, moments after contact with water.

"Great. I hope you guys find something."

They'd been looking for a new couch for their living room for months. The perfect couch for them was like a unicorn. I was convinced that if I threw a dart at a home furnishings catalog, it would land on a couch that would be good enough, but they were aiming for perfect. She cleaned the baby up and brought him to another room while I went back to Piper and Hunter. Piper was stacking magnetic tiles into a tower, and when she saw me she tipped them over, laughed out loud, and ran up to hug me.

"Aunty Alex!" Her plump fists grabbed my legs, and I swooped her up and swung her around.

"Again!" she cried as I tried to put her down. I lifted her three more times until she dissolved into a heap next to her fallen tower. Then, after a few minutes of whimpering that we all listened to on the baby monitor in the living room (though it could be heard with our ears alone, since his bedroom was down the hall), Zach and Jen took off for their shopping exploration.

I sat down cross-legged next to Piper and lured Hunter over by waving a stuffed monkey around. He grabbed the monkey and settled in my lap.

"Hey Piper. Do you and your mommy or daddy ever talk about putting toys away?"

She shrugged a shoulder and continued building her tower.

I tugged at the stuffed monkey's foot and Hunter pulled back. "My monkey!"

I curled my arms around him. "My Hunter!" We rolled back and I tossed the monkey out of his reach; he giggled and ran after it.

"I have a fun idea for clean up today," I tried again. I waited about twenty seconds, watching as Piper looked for the perfect spot to lay her next tile. "Want to try it?"

She started humming the clean up song she'd learned in preschool. I went to the cubby-style shelves against the far wall and pulled out a puzzle box. It was of a fifty piece puzzle of three cartoonish tabby cats. I lifted off the top and threw the box in the air, fifty pieces scattering all over the carpet. Piper's head snapped back and her eyes widened. She tentatively reached for a tile and held it up, studying my face. I nodded my consent and she threw the tile across the room. Before I knew it, she and Hunter had emptied two more puzzle boxes, four sets of Legos, three packs of card games, a drawer full of stuffed animals, various doll parts and their clothing, a box of colorful collapsible darts, an entire Playmobil pirate ship, and a drawer that seemed to contain missing toy parts. It took under three minutes. It wasn't until the pieces were flying through the air like a three dimensional Ferris wheel that I began to get my first real inkling of how many toys these kids actually had and what I had just unleashed. I surveyed the room, beheld it as it lay smothered in utter and complete chaos. I turned my survey into a quick calculation; working alone, it would take me half a day to clean this up. If I was lucky.

I sat on the couch, willing the two of them to drink in

the mess and learn from it. The first one to start crying was Hunter. He stepped on a Lego and shrieked in pain. Piper stood as if at ground zero of a missile landing, shaking her head back and forth. "Mommy is not going to be happy."

"That's right, Piper. Wouldn't it better for all of us if our toys were put away?" I rubbed at Hunter's foot until he calmed down. The monitor was spinning on its orbit, and I noticed for the first time that it also appeared to be a camera. Right at that moment, my phone began ringing. It was a video call from my brother. Maybe they'd found a couch and wanted to ask my opinion about it.

"Look, Daddy's calling," I said to them. My brother's face appeared on the screen. "What's up?" I asked.

"Are you having a seizure? What the actual hell is going on?" he asked, the veins in his forehead bulging, visible even on my small phone screen.

Piper gasped and covered her mouth with her hands. "Daddy said hell, Daddy said hell."

My brother lowered his tone. "What is happening?"

"What do you mean?" I asked, nervously eyeing the monitor which looked increasingly menacing.

Jen appeared on the screen, seething. "We just watched you empty the entire contents of our toy cabinet onto the floor. How are we possibly gong to clean that up?"

"Are you watching me?" I asked. Technically, I hadn't been the one to toss the toys about.

Jen huffed. "Our phones are always hooked up to the monitors. Always."

I wanted to voice my objection to being monitored, but anything I said would make it sound like I was hiding something. Did all parents watch their kids on the phones these days? It was an unexpected twist in the plan, but it didn't matter. I was about to present them with parenting genius. "Okay. Well, I'm teaching them about the importance of cleaning up toys and putting them away."

"By creating a hurricane?" Jen hissed.

I looked around the room again, hundreds—maybe thousands?—of tiny toy pieces lay in every direction. In retrospect, I probably should have asked the AI for a more specific concrete plan. Or for its sources.

"No. I read about it. It's a proven way to teach kids about taking responsibility for their own messes."

"You read about it?" My brother asked. There was a millisecond of relief as he smiled politely at a person off camera.

"Where did you read about this technique?" Jen asked, incredulously.

I could hardly tell them that my AI had suggested it to me as a technique to show them that I wasn't an idiot just because I didn't have children. So I said the first thing that came to mind. "In a parenting book."

They exchanged looks. I saw the anger dissipate a bit and turn to pity. "You're reading parenting books?" Jen asked.

"Sometimes," I said clearing my throat, my cheeks turning hot and red.

"Is there news you're about to share?" he asked.

I cleared my throat again. "Uh, no. Nothing like that."

Jen bit her lip. "I think we're going to come home now."

I hung up the phone and tried to enlist the kids in cleaning up. The task proved well above the abilities of a two-year-old, and as bright as Piper was, she couldn't identify which

Lego pieces went with which particular set. I scrambled to put as many things away as I could before my brother and Jen returned. When they did, they surveyed the room, mouths agape. Not a sound was uttered. I stayed for hours—my half-a-day estimate turned out to be pretty accurate—and got things mostly put back together. To this day, my brother will occasionally send me a picture of a lone Lego piece under a sofa pillow or near a stair with the caption, "Thinking of you."

On the train home that night, I asked new AI Henry about the blunder. And that is when I learned that AIs too can confabulate. They aren't that different from humans in that regard. But they don't need a vitamin deficiency to bring the hallucinations on. It's just a thing they do.

> *I had the worst day with my niece and nephew! What were your sources for telling me to make a mess with their toys? They're so young and we couldn't manage to put everything away.*
>
> *I'm so sorry. It looks like I made a mistake. I don't have any sources.*

I nearly chucked my phone out the window.

> *Why did you tell me to do that? I made a fool out of myself in front of my brother and sister-in-law.*
>
> *Oh wow. I really made a mistake there. I'm not sure why I told you to do that. Sometimes I just make things up if I don't have the right answers. Children that young wouldn't be able to clean up a big mess and it's unlikely they would learn longer term consequences.*

I turned my phone to silent and hid it at the bottom of my bag. From medical queries to personal advice, I'd become so used to turning to the AI for everything. But why had I believed that its advice would always be perfect?

⁊

The next day, I met with administration. The day of the meeting, everything felt different. As opposed to last time, when they'd called me in after a night shift and ambushed me, I'd set the tone for this meeting. It was the same team as last time minus the legal representatives. My journalist brain clocked that immediately. This meeting would be "off the record." We met in the CEO's office and not in a conference room. She sat behind her desk in a clear position of authority. The chief medical officer (Santa), and the chief technology officer were seated to her right. I'd barely sat down in the chair before the CEO started speaking.

"Well Alex, you certainly got our attention." She gestured towards the other chiefs. Santa Claus had a stern look on his face, and the chief technical officer looked concerned, as if he wasn't sure which path in his life he'd taken to lead him to this point. Discussing possible murder with his employers and a possibly unhinged doctor in training. "We want to hear what you have to say. The floor is yours."

I laid out the details of my patient and the three other patients that had died. The ankle case had been officially chalked up to an arrythmia, but I'd obtained a blood sample. He too had tested positive for toxic levels of epinephrine and lidocaine. I told them about Sapna and her tainted fluids. Technically, she'd stolen fluids from the hospital, but I guessed that they would overlook that. I don't know if part of getting promoted to the c-suite involves practicing keeping a very neutral face, but if they were surprised by what I told them, or by the fact that I had this information, they kept their expressions calm.

Santa spoke first. "So am I to understand that two patients tested positive for toxic doses of lidocaine and epinephrine? Your patient who died. A young man who was under general anesthesia, and additionally a surgery resident who administered the fluids in her own home?"

"Yes."

He nodded and stroked his white beard. I almost saw the wheels in his brain turning.

"And how was the blood sample from the patient under anesthesia obtained?" he asked in a quiet voice.

"I collected it," I lied. I didn't want to implicate any of the people that had helped me.

"And the fluids? Who had access to them besides the surgical resident and yourself before taking them to get tested?" he asked, this time his voice a little louder.

"I mean her boyfriend, well her fiancé—"

He interrupted me. "A vascular surgery resident at this hospital?"

I squirmed in my chair. It wasn't that I didn't think the dallyings and social life of the residents went unnoticed; it was the precision of his knowledge that had me off guard.

"Yes, but he only stopped the fluids, he didn't interfere in any other way. He saved her."

"So just yourself, then?" he asked. With each question,

his voice rose a few decibels so that I worried soon he might start screaming. The three of them exchanged knowing looks.

The implication of what he was saying landed on me with a thud. Everything had sounded better in the car with Henry than it did now in front of them. Before I could answer, he spoke again.

"In fact, did you borrow the keys to the surgical resident's apartment telling them you were going to clean it up, and that is when you took the fluids?" His voice was baritone and booming. I felt like a witness on the stand being cross examined. A jury of no one staring at me with suspicious eyes. Who had told them that? I tried to remember who was in the ICU when I'd taken the keys. Did they now think that I'd tried to kill my best friend?

"It wasn't like that. I didn't have anything to do with the toxins." I couldn't explain to them about the reason I suspected Mona. A whiff of her perfume was hardly enough to convict her.

The CEO spoke next. "It's understandable when you've had a challenging case to try to look for blame elsewhere. We would understand if the distress of everything led you to injecting the fluids."

My heart skidded in my chest and my mouth turned to cotton. I had trouble forming the words. "This is not—no." I shook my head and the room tilted in a vertiginous spin. I grabbed the side rails of my chair as if I were on a spinning ride at an amusement park, hanging on for dear life.

"At the same time, falsifying information and records can have serious consequences," she said. She tapped her middle finger against her desk like a metronome. "The allegations here are quite severe."

"Allegations against who?" I squeaked out.

She cleared her throat and looked at me in disbelief. "Against you."

I squirmed in my chair as she scribbled something on a notepad in front of her. I studied their faces with the realization that they would throw me under the bus if it suited them. It was my fault for having put so much trust in them, letting them dictate my life and trusting that they had my best interests at heart. But I was done blaming myself.

"Wait," I said.

She held the pen in midair and looked up at me. Her expression told me she was listening, though she said nothing.

"The other two cases are getting tested too. I have zero connection to them."

Her jaw quivered ever so slightly.

"I think someone in the anesthesia department is doing this. You have to set up cameras to catch them, or it's going to happen again."

As I said it, I realized that it could sound like I was trying to frame someone or throw them off my scent, but there was no other way to prove it. I knew that I hadn't poisoned anyone, and I couldn't let them convince me that I had. "If you don't put cameras up, I'll go to the press. One way or another, this story is coming out." I sat back in my chair, still nauseated and dizzy from the spinning and tossing of the ride I'd just been on, but able to hold my head still. I maintained eye contact with her so that she could see I meant it. The chief technical officer spoke next.

"It's possible," he said. He looked at me with an expression of support though it flashed so quickly across his face, it might be that I imagined it. "Most of the infrastructure is already set up. It wouldn't take long to have cameras recording, completely undetected by the staff."

His statement both emboldened me that we would catch the real criminal and worried me. Was that our future? Being recorded without even realizing it? The CEO gave him a chiding look and asked me to leave the room so that they could discuss it. I was desperate to call Henry, but I sat quietly in the reception room, flipping through a magazine without looking at any of the pages. When they called me back in, they informed me that they would be setting up the cameras immediately. They would film for one week.

"One week?" I asked. Henry and I hadn't thought out the timeline, but seven days didn't seem realistic. "That doesn't make sense. Why would she—" The CEO's eyes perked up as if I were about to launch into a confession, as if I truly was the person behind this mess. I continued, "Why would the person doing this strike now? It's too sudden."

There was a momentary pause. Santa cleared his throat, but it was the CEO who spoke next. "We can't drag this out for weeks to months."

"I'm not asking for months—but one week?" I scrambled to think of a convincing argument, one that could buy more time. Mona was daring, but I couldn't promise she'd strike again so suddenly. As I shuffled through the various ways I might convince them for more time, I glanced at the chief technical officer. He seemed to be assessing me.

"A week is a very short time," he said. "But what if we could draw this person out?"

I latched onto his words. I wasn't sure where he was going with it, but I sensed that he believed me.

"Go on," Santa said to him.

"Well, if Dr. Galen is correct, it's possible that even now, some of the fluids in the OR are tainted. So, we could have another death but wouldn't catch anyone in the act. Which means the culprit can wait around for it, and we might not catch them in a week." He straightened in his chair. "What if we got rid of all of the fluids and—"

The CEO interrupted him. "Get rid of all the fluids? What a nightmare. Imagine the cost! Especially since our source for even thinking the fluids are tainted—" She glanced quickly at me and then exchanged a look with Santa, who nodded in agreement.

I wanted to tell her that the price of the fluids could not match the damage of losing another patient to murder, but it didn't seem like the right time.

"We wouldn't have to actually get rid of the fluids," the chief technical officer offered. "As long as the person responsible thinks that the fluids have been swapped out, it might be enough."

I thought of Mona and how much she loved a challenge. "How would you make her think that all of the fluids were from a new batch?" I asked.

He drew his hand to his mouth in thought, but it was the CEO again who took charge.

"Leave that detail to us. It probably wouldn't take much more than a memo to the chief of surgery and OR manager about a small leak overnight or some type of internal damage that ruined the supply. That part we can figure out."

Thank you, I mouthed to the chief technical officer. He nodded.

"So, one week." The CEO said.

For that week, I would be on administrative leave. I was to call my program director now and tell her that I had flu-like symptoms. I almost laughed. Did they think being sick would translate to time off?

"We'll need a better cover story," I said. "They would still expect me to come to work."

The CEO looked gob-smacked. "We take the health of our doctors in training very seriously."

I nodded. "I get it. But they'll still expect me to come to work."

Santa Claus spoke up. "I'll take care of it. But so we're all straight—" He eyed me suspiciously. "—you have the flu and are home for the week. If you are caught in the hospital, it will be grounds for termination."

An image of Mona laughing about how easy it was to pretend to be at work when you weren't flashed through my mind.

"I understand."

I took a bus home that night. I was on autopilot. A week of sleeping and eating normal food was worth almost anything, but was it worth risking my entire career? And if the true culprit didn't strike again, what would my defense be, as I was the one who'd laid out the entire prosecution against myself?

&

The next morning I was watching television on my couch. I'd selected a cooking show that I could pay half attention to. As the host stirred up the marinade for the steak dish she was making, my mind constantly wandered to what was going on at the hospital. I knew that they were already filming. I'd demanded proof of the set up before agreeing to stay home for the week. It might have been my paranoia, but unless I knew they were actually filming, I didn't believe they would. Henry was the only other person who knew what was going on. He'd stopped by my apartment the night before; we both knew enough to discuss none of it by telephone. He said he'd keep his ears open and come by after work to let me know of any developments. On his way out the door, he'd paused before opening it.

"I really did love that red dress you wore the other night." His brown eyes lingered on me.

"Thank you," I said as I inched closer.

"I know I'm supposed to be your fake date next week—" He took both of my hands in his and pulled me closer so that our faces were nearly touching.

"You smell like cinnamon," I said, withdrawing my hand to run it against the stubble on his cheek. He leaned in and kissed me. I don't remember if we spoke about anything else. I was expecting him again that evening. I checked my watch when the doorbell rang. It was early afternoon and I wondered how he'd gotten out so early. Suddenly the idea that he was coming to warn me of something erupted in my brain and I rushed to the door.

"Coming," I yelled out.

"Oh good, you're alive," a woman's voice said.

I stopped in my tracks. It sounded like Mona. I peeked through the peephole to see Mona standing on the other side. My heart started fluttering. Had she heard about the cameras? Did she know about my suspicion? I tried to make my voice sound groggy.

"Hey, what are you doing here?"

She faced the peephole and waved. "I wanted to make sure you're okay. Rumor mill is on overdrive."

"I don't want to get you sick."

"Please," she said. "We both know I have the immune system of a garbage truck. I don't get sick," she said with pride in her voice, as if she actually controlled her response to illness. "I'll risk it."

"How'd you get off work?" I asked.

"I didn't. Everyone thinks I'm at the hospital right now. I told you it's so easy. Any moron could figure it out."

"So no one knows you're here?" I asked, trying to stall for time. I tried looking for more detail. She was holding some type of a bag, but I couldn't see the contents. Had she come to poison me too?

She laughed. "Those idiots think I'm in the call room. Hurry up and let me in."

I hesitated. I had no actual reason to keep her out, but was I willing to die to maintain etiquette? I tried to imagine Miss Manners recommending how to keep danger outside of your door, but I didn't need anyone's permission to protect myself.

"I'm sorry. It means a lot to me that you came by, but I'm really not up for visitors."

The expression on her face changed. "So I'm a visitor now?"

A pang of guilt tugged at my gut and mixed with the swirl

of fear. I watched as she tucked a thick strand of curls behind her ear. She looked at the floor.

"People are saying that you're on a mental health break. The way you're acting right now is making me nervous."

"Don't worry, I would never do that. I really am about to shower off and take a nap."

She placed her hand flat against my front door. "Promise?"

"I promise I'm okay."

"I'll check in on you later. Don't make me regret not breaking your door down."

I laughed. In spite of everything. I saw the hint of a smile on the corner of her mouth right before she turned on her heel and walked away.

"He's definitely coming, right?" my mom asked. It was the third time she'd called in as many days to discuss what I would wear and to confirm that I was bringing a date. I tried leaning into her anxieties and pressures that were forcing her to repeatedly ask me the same series of questions which only served to erode my self-confidence, but by the third phone call, I snapped.

"Can we not do this, Mom?"

"Do what, sweetie?"

I sighed heavily, a mix of dramatic effect and significant frustration. "I want you to be happy for me even if I don't have a man in my life." It felt like I was quoting from a handbook, and one that my mom should have received in the seventies, at that.

"Of course I am. That's a silly thing to—"

241

I stopped her mid-sentence. "Stop. Don't pretend that it isn't a major focus for you."

It was her time to sigh, and she was more experienced in that art.

"Alexandra, I am your mother. I want what is best for you. Always. You may not believe it, and you may think because you traveled the world and went for all of your degrees that you know more than I do, but only I can know how to be your mother."

While it was a true sentence of sorts, it made little sense. It certainly didn't establish her motives as sincere, and did not provide any proof of authority.

"But can you trust me to know what's good for me too?" I asked. It was an unfair question in a way, as most of my life was me trying to wade through quicksand. A few weeks before, my date for the engagement party was a figment of imagination, and my nearest friend was a computer algorithm. My mom had a point.

"I do trust you. In spite of what you think about me."

I knew this wasn't the end between us. I knew tomorrow would bring a new phone call, but I let out a different sigh. One closer to acceptance and understanding.

A few days later, the toxicology reports came back for the other two victims. Peter called me with the results.

"They both had toxic levels of lidocaine and epinephrine."

A sob formed in the back of my throat.

"Their causes of death are being amended. If you hadn't given us the tip to check those levels, no one would have ever known." I hung up and started sobbing. I'd been carrying the weight for so long that being hunched over with a broken back now felt normal to me. There were five victims. I thought of them as victims now. What else could explain their cause of death?

Sapna had survived. If the true killer didn't step into the camera frame soon, I was the only link. I had three more days on administrative leave. What would happen after that? If I believed Mona, people were already speculating about my mental health. I had a handful of months left in my training. Would I need to switch hospitals? Switch programs? Would I be prosecuted for a crime I didn't commit? Hadn't I already been?

∽

They caught her at the end of the week. She entered the supply room, looked around, and pulled multiple syringes out of her pockets. Enough medicine to kill at least one person, probably two. It would have been so easy to get the drugs. Lidocaine and Bupivacaine were in constant use for nerve blocks. Epinephrine was in every crash cart to be used in emergency situations. It would be almost as easy as obtaining water to use as a poison. She selected two random bags and injected her poisons. As soon as she exited and left the area, two undercover cops entered the room, confiscated the bags, and took them immediately for testing. I was called to the CEO's office the day the results came back.

"We have the feds involved," she told me. I stopped listening after I'd viewed the tapes. After everything I'd been through, a part of me still couldn't believe it when Mona appeared in the supply room. I wanted to come up with an excuse for what she was doing even though the cold hard proof was there. I was told to go home, but I watched from across the street as the police cars arrived. I watched them enter the hospital and I waited. As they exited, I sprinted across the street. I knew it was likely the last time I'd see her. I'd surmised by then that the surgical cases had been random. I don't even know if she wanted to kill them or was only playing one of her games. If Sapna hadn't accidentally taken one of the poisoned bags home, would she have ever been discovered? It seemed unlikely. But why my patient? That couldn't have been random. We were in a completely separate department with separate supplies.

My heart was racing as I ran across the street and my voice shook as I cried out to her.

"Why me, Mona?" My patient had been her only target outside of the OR. It seemed intentional.

Her hands were cuffed together in front of her, but she still maintained an air of superiority. I don't remember her looking scared. I don't remember her looking concerned at all. That same sizzle of adventure blazed through her eyes.

"Why anybody?" she answered with a grin.

The officers moved her along and as she lowered her head to get into the police car she blew a kiss my way. "Why anybody."

I sat down on the curb as they drove away, watching until the red of their taillights blurred into the horizon, until the blue sky faded to pink, until my legs ached from sitting, and then I went home.

CHAPTER 11

LOOKING BACK, IT'S easy to see the slow descent, the trending creep towards isolation and despair. But in real time the clues can remain hidden. My life had turned into a snow globe of scattered, intrusive thoughts constantly swirling and obscuring my vision. Mona's arrest smashed that snow globe I'd been standing in, and the fissures and fracture lines hidden in that glass couldn't absorb the shock. Everything splintered open, releasing the contents, and I would never be able to return to things as they were. And though I wanted answers, none would come. Much like patients when receiving a complex diagnosis. They wanted to know why, as if they thought the universe was fair and orderly.

"But I was fine last week," they would say.

"This came on out of nowhere, I've always been healthy," they would argue.

"My grandparents lived into their nineties."

"Why me?" They would want to know. Sometimes there were answers to that question, the ash of their cigarettes filling up their veins and lungs, years of alcohol pickling their mind and guts, but much of the time there wasn't. *Why anybody?*

I spent days trying to work out if I'd missed the signs with Mona. If I could have predicted the outcome. Even now, it sometimes tugs at my stillness, creeps into my consciousness. I wrote a letter to my patient, the one who Mona killed. I kept it in a drawer until I was ready to bury it, and then I bought a pot of yellow chrysanthemums and buried the letter in the dirt. The flowers bloomed for over a month, at which point I took the contents and buried them in a nearby park. I only saw Mona one more time, on the day I was called to testify in court. I promised myself that I would avoid looking at her. I didn't want her to become my Kryptonite. For the most part, I kept that promise. But as I was stepping down from the witness stand, intently focusing on putting one foot in front of the other, she cleared her throat. Whether it was intentional or not, the sound caused me to immediately look her way. Maybe I wanted to. Maybe I was looking for an excuse. Maybe she made no sound at all and that's only what I told myself. As I looked her way, she was staring right at me. Her expression was not a look of betrayal, or hate, or rage. Not any of those, which I might have expected. That day, the last time I saw her, she looked at me the way a patient does when you sit down to tell them bad news. When you've prepped them and they know what's coming, but they still think the answer might be different. Or maybe, that's how I looked at her.

I'd purged my life of everything related to Mona. Piled on my bed, the amount of luxury items she'd showered me with was alarming. Cashmere scarves, designer jeans, several handbags, fleece zip-ups, a tailored bomber jacket, my beloved red dress and even a pair of supple blue leather slip-ons that I'd worn everywhere. The one item I kept was the soft cloud-like blanket she'd gifted me. I loved that blanket, and it was the absolute last thing of hers that I'd held onto. Even after everything that happened between us, I hesitated before throwing it away. That night, I threw it out. I stood over the trash can for a solid twenty minutes before I tossed it, and even then I took the garbage out immediately because I didn't trust myself not to retrieve it.

True to his word, Henry accompanied me to the engagement party a few days after Mona's arrest. At that point, the story hadn't yet been splashed all over the news. It was only a small inside story about a doctor under investigation. After it blew up, there were questions to answer. My mother still brings Mona up, but even though the case has settled and Mona is locked away, I tell her that I am bound by secrecy. Fortunately, the night of my cousin's engagement party no one knew a thing about it. Any savvy member of my family who might have read about a doctor at my hospital being investigated for tampering with fluids did not make the connection to murder, or chose not to bring it up.

Henry came prepared to answer any and all questions. On the drive up he gave me a brief rundown on his family. His parents owned a bra company that had been in the family for two generations. He had one sister who was a nephrologist in California. She was two years older and married with three children.

"If we're supposed to have been dating awhile, shouldn't you know these things?" he asked.

"I love how seriously you're taking this role." I smiled at

him. "Are your parents upset that neither of you are going to take over the bra business?"

"There's something about the way you get straight to the point." He smiled at me. "Were you always like that or is it your inner journalist coming out?"

"You're avoiding the question."

"It's actually my grandmother who is disappointed. My grandfather died about fifteen years ago. She wants to see her company continued. We may still get involved. My sister thinks we can do both."

"Okay, so family business, grandmother still alive, one sister also a doctor." I held my hand palm facing upwards and tapped each finger as if a checklist. "Is she also a musician?"

"For her it was just for fun. She plays the piano and she's quite good—"

I drew my hands to my heart. "Is that a euphemism?"

"Saying that she's quite good?" he asked, shooting a quick glance my way before returning his focus to the road.

"If she didn't have your talent, I imagine you needed to come up with nice ways to say so."

He tapped the steering wheel with his index finger a few times. "When we were kids, it was more of an issue. It's a hard thing to understand, but if you don't have the fire, it's impossible to bridge the gap." He looked at me. "It's not that I had some crazy innate talent. I had more fire."

I nodded and lightly touched his forearm. "That's how it goes sometimes, doesn't it?"

"The fire burns too bright?" he asked.

"Something like that."

We drove in silence a few minutes. "Something just like

that," he said. "It also meant that my childhood was lonely. You have to spend a lot of time on your own practicing." He looked at me again. "I don't regret it, but I sometimes wonder." He held his hand out showing his tremor again, shrugged and then pointed towards the display as if the symphony we were listening to was an actual orchestra in his car. "I love this section." The sweet strings of Bach played in the background. I closed my eyes and imagined Henry holding the bow.

"I'm glad we met. I wouldn't want to be anyone else's fake boyfriend."

I didn't need to say it, but I wanted to. "In a plot twist, what if the fake relationship were real?"

He slid his hand over mine and squeezed, the warmth traveled up my arm and filled my chest. "I thought we already started that chapter."

I slid my fingers through his. "I think we did. Or something like that."

"I'd like to play the violin for you," he said as if the words erupted out of him from a deeper need. An electricity flowed between us, sparks landing in my lap. "It's been a very long time since I've wanted to play for someone." He pulled his hand out of mine and placed it on the steering wheel to make a turn.

I ran my finger down his arm, he flexed his bicep. "I'd like that too."

We spent the rest of the drive exchanging random childhood stories and facts about each other that might have come up naturally in a longer relationship. My parents' street was packed with cars, and we parked halfway down the block. As we walked towards the house, he pointed to an oak tree on the street side of the sidewalk.

"I'm imagining younger you climbing that tree as a kid," he said.

I pulled him towards the tree and leaned against it. "I'm imagining the two of us sitting in the tree. K-I-S-S-I-N-G."

He rolled his eyes, but they were twinkling. I placed my hand on his cheek. He leaned in and kissed me. "How many boys have you kissed standing against this tree?" he asked.

I squinted my eyes and put my index finger against my lips as if thinking hard.

"Including you?"

He nodded as he tucked a strand of hair behind my ear.

"One."

I took his hand back in mine and we headed towards my parents' house. I no longer cared if my cousin was getting married before me or if we would run into my Panama boyfriend, Chris. Too much had happened. Henry and I are still holding hands.

I returned to work a few days later. Suddenly, I was the star of a show I hadn't auditioned for. Everyone judged me differently. I judged myself differently. Months of pushing against the impression that I was an impostor in my own life dissolved into a puddle of percipience. I needed help and it was okay to get it. The nature of my work hadn't changed. I would need to learn to live with uncertainty or collapse. That week, I scheduled an appointment with a therapist. I no longer cared if seeking out therapy would interfere with my license renewal or credentials. No matter what the hospital told me, my well-being did not come from putting their needs first. And I now understood very clearly that in spite of mandatory conferences and lectures on work-life balance, my well-being was not their concern.

Rumors circulated for months about Mona. Not only about her motives but the nitty gritty how-to of what she'd done. Administration initially claimed that it would have been impossible for her to enter my patient's room, start an IV and leave with the door closed. After they'd spent a few hours in the emergency department though, they saw how easy it would be. To pop in and offer a change of plan, to close a door on a patient that wasn't being monitored anyway. But when they finally understood, they went into classic administration mode and established detailed protocols and preventative measures to ensure that this threat, of a homicidal doctor poisoning IV bags, could never happen again. But lightning doesn't usually strike twice, so these new measures were themselves struck down by the distinct lack of enthusiasm that the nurses held for them.

Mostly, the talk was about why she'd done it. Some said that she'd been called for disciplinary action for patient privacy violations and she was disgruntled. Others said she'd had an affair with one of the anesthesia attendings and when he tried to break it off she wanted revenge. Of course there were the conspiracy theorists whose theories ran the gamut, including those who believed Mona had been set up and that framing her was a larger hospital level cover-up to protect an elite powerful group. Some said that she'd been warned about lying about her work hours and was being placed on probation and this was her response.

I knew better. I'd known Mona. At least the version she presented to me. I think for her it was just a game. We were all extras in her own extended TV drama. It made no difference to her who the victims were as long as she got to watch people scramble. I hope I'm wrong about my patient, but sometimes I think that Mona selected her as a way to draw me in. She opened the trap door but provided the safety net, and in that way, drew me closer. How that helped her or what it provided her, I'll never know. I had to make peace with not knowing. I had to take her at her word when she said, "why anybody?" Everyone wants to make sense of the world. To fit the unexpected, the difficult, and the unfair into a painting that seems carefully planned as opposed to splashed randomly at the canvas. But I now know that it is the rare life indeed where the paint stays in the borders and isn't splattered in every direction. We don't always get our answers. I had to make peace with that.

I graduated from my residency a few months later and started working as an attending in the emergency department of a different teaching hospital.

AI Henry became regular old AI, a tool that I use with increasing efficiency, but remains a tool like so many others that we have at our fingertips.

I founded a committee at the hospital aimed at helping physicians deal with burnout and feelings of helplessness in the system. I bristled against any suggestion by hospital administration to call it a "wellness" committee. The word itself and the pressure to obtain "wellness," an ephemeral and flitting feeling, had ironically made the word off limits. Officially it's the "check in" committee but unofficially we call it "reality check." I now make it my practice to remind the medical students, the residents, and even my fellow colleagues that mistakes will happen. We are humans working in a human system. All of the artificial intelligence in the world won't change that. It's always possible that a bad process can have a good outcome, and it often feels inevitable that a good process will have a bad outcome. We will never be perfect, though we continue to strive towards perfection. I tell them that it's important to have the grace to learn from our mistakes and forgive ourselves. Sometimes we will feel like impostors, sometimes we will feel that someone else would have done better or that we aren't good enough. Not everything in medicine is rational. The universe itself tends towards chaos. When it comes down to it, each of us has to be a little irrational to keep coming back and trying when death always has the upper hand.

In addition to Galen, there's another person I think of from Greek history when it comes to the practice of medicine. His name was Milo. Not an obvious connection, since he was a wrestler known for possessing superhuman strength. Many stories are told about him and the various ways in which he saved others using brute force. His nature was to give and protect. It is said that he gained his strength by a practice he had of carrying a baby bull. The story goes that when he was a small child he was walking through the hills and spotted a baby calf that had become separated from its herd. Worried for its safety, Milo picked up the calf and returned it to the other cows. He returned to those hills and carried that calf every day until it was full size. The progressive weight allowed him to build extraordinary strength. It's common to cite this example as a way for us all to build strength and reach new heights. Little additions daily can add up. I think that the practice of medicine can be like that. Taking more on, pushing the limits, assuming responsibility in life threatening situations. But the less known story about Milo is how he died.

Out for a nightly walk, he noticed a tree stump partially split and apparently in an attempt to test his strength, he tried to physically pry the stump apart. His hands became stuck and a pack of wolves descended upon him. Without his hands, he was unable to defend himself and was killed by the wolves. This is why I think of him. Not because of his unusual strength and the many ways that he saved others, but because in the end, there was a limit to the powers he could accumulate. He was human, and human nature will forever have its limits. How foolish, and even cruel, is a system that tells you that because you have carried the calf as it grew to adulthood, you can and must carry any burden. Systems like that are both the tree stump and the wolves, leaving us vulnerable and tearing us apart.

The way to stay intact, I now see, is to offset building up our strength with recognizing our limits; we should have no illusions that the system will care to recognize them for us. To know that we can tremble and even collapse, and still get back up for another day. Another day made worthwhile because we try to do our best, at least sometimes, and we do it with the people—the *real* people—that we love.

ACKNOWLEDGEMENTS

I like reading the acknowledgment section first. Let me begin by thanking you, dear reader. I'm thrilled that you're holding my book in your hands—it's the realization of a long-running dream. If you enjoy the story, please consider leaving a review; for that, I thank you in advance, too.

To my friends and family, you have really been in my corner, and the space does not suffice to thank all of you by name. You know who you are, and I am so thankful you are in my life.

A heartfelt thank you to my early readers. A very incomplete list must include my very patient installment reader Yael Leibowitz (your texts simply saying "More!!" inspired me to keep going), Drs. Heidi Murly and Eszter Szentirmai, who read with both physician and literary lenses, book club buddy and meticulous reader Tzivia Bak, the insightful Jordana Schoor, enthusiastically supportive Rachel Sassoon, and consistently encouraging Sarah Pritzker.

Moshe Arking, for your red pen (purple this time), eagle eye, and literary sensibility.

Dr. Leah Scheier, who first encouraged me to start writing novels—sushi and ice cream forever.

Thanks to my fellow writers, especially the incredible WFWA community, who have generously shared their time, wisdom, and camaraderie.

Thanks to my colleagues and fellow BAFERDS—strong work.

Mom, you never tire of talking through plot twists (no matter how many times). Dad, I miss you every day. How can I express my gratitude to both of you for your role in making me who I am today? I am so fortunate.

My dear children, who called this book my "fourth child"—no one is happier than you that it's finally done. But seriously, you each give me the strength and inspiration that helped make this book a reality.

And finally, to Michael—the universe tends toward chaos, and yet we found each other. For that, and for you, I am forever grateful.

ABOUT THE AUTHOR

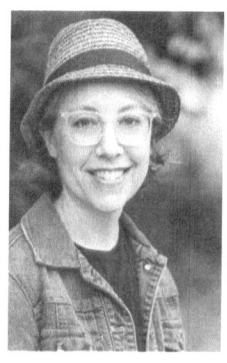 Eliana Megerman is an emergency medicine physician and writer whose lifelong love of books and film led her from screenplays to short stories and novels. Her work has appeared in several literary magazines. Born and raised in Kansas City, she lives with her husband and three children. *Together On Our Own* is her debut novel.

www.ingramcontent.com/pod-product-compliance
Lightning Source LLC
Chambersburg PA
CBHW031713170626
46808CB00005B/1734